CW01395135

Psychology
in
Progress

General editor: Peter Herriot

Aspects
of
Psychopharmacology

Psychology in Progress

Already available

Aspects
of
Psychopharmacology

edited by
D. J. SANGER
and
D. E. BLACKMAN

METHUEN
London and New York

First published in 1984 by
Methuen & Co. Ltd
11 New Fetter Lane, London EC4P 4EE

Published in the USA by
Methuen & Co.
in association with Methuen, Inc.
733 Third Avenue, New York, NY 10017

Typeset by Scarborough Typesetting Services
and printed in Great Britain by
Richard Clay (The Chaucer Press), Ltd
Bungay, Suffolk

British Library Cataloguing in Publication Data

Aspects of psychopharmacology. —(Psychology
in Progress)
1. Psychopharmacology
I. Sanger, D.J. II. Blackman, D.E.
III. Series
615'.78 RC483

ISBN 0−416−33940−9
ISBN 0−416−33950−6 Pbk

Contents

Notes on the contributors

James E. Barrett is Associate Professor of Psychiatry, Medical Psychology and Pharmacology at the Uniformed Services University of the Health Sciences, Bethesda, Maryland, USA. His research interests have concentrated on the analysis of operant behaviour and on determinants of the behavioural effects of drugs.

Derek Blackman is Professor and Head of the Department of Psychology at University College, Cardiff. He was President of the British Psychological Society in 1981/2, and is currently editor of the *British Journal of Psychology*. His principal interests are contemporary behaviourism, especially operant conditioning, and psychopharmacology. He is the author of *Operant Conditioning* (Methuen, 1974), and co-editor with D. J. Sanger of *Contemporary Research in Behavioral Pharmacology* (Plenum, 1978).

Raymond Cochrane is Senior Lecturer and Head of the Department of Psychology at the University of Birmingham. He has written extensively on the social psychology of social problems and mental illness. His most recent book is *The Social Creation of Mental Illness* (Longman, 1983). His research interests have been focused on the way in which immigrants adjust to life in a new country and the consequences of migration for mental health. In addition he has recently been involved in studies of the development of political awareness in adolescents and of ways to increase the effectiveness of police–community relations.

Andrew Greenshaw is a Postdoctoral Fellow at the Psychiatric Research Division of the University of Saskatchewan, Canada. He is Language Editor for the international journal *General Physiology and Biophysics*. His research interests focus on the behavioural effects of electrical and chemical stimulation of the brain, particularly in the context of instrumental and classical conditioning. At present he is (with Dr C. T. Dourish) editing a book on behavioural approaches to the analysis of drug effects.

P. E. Harrison-Read is currently Registrar in Psychiatry at St Mary's Hospital, London. He was formerly Lecturer in Pharmacology at St Bartholomew's Hospital Medical College, London. His main research interests are in the behavioural pharmacology of lithium and anti-depressant drugs.

Geoff Lowe is Senior Lecturer in Psychology at Hull University and has published articles on various aspects of both human and animal psychopharmacology. He is especially interested in the use of drugs as tools in the investigation of behaviour. His early work was concerned with attempts to develop drug-induced models (in animals) of behavioural abnormality. His current research interests centre on the psychopharmacology of alcohol, including state-dependent learning, alcohol-stress interactions, and the mechanisms (and modifying factors) of alcohol intoxication.

David J. Sanger is Project Leader in charge of behavioural research at Laboratoires d'Etudes et de Recherches Synthelabo, a French pharmaceutical company situated south of Paris. After obtaining a first degree in psychology and physiology from Nottingham University he carried out research and obtained a Ph.D. from the Pharmacology Department of University College, London. He has worked as an ICI Research Fellow in the University of Birmingham, a Lecturer in Psychology at University College, Cardiff and a Senior Section Leader in the Pharmacology Department of Reckitt and Colman. His present work involves behavioural research with animals aimed at the discovery and evaluation of new and better psychoactive drugs.

Christine Smith is Lecturer in Pharmacology at the London Hospital Medical College, London. Her research interests currently are the nature of cognitive disorder in Alzheimer's disease and the role of the central cholinergic system in memory processes.

Ian Stolerman is at the Institute of Psychiatry, University of London as a member of the UK Medical Research Council's scientific staff. His research is primarily concerned with conditioned behaviour in animal subjects and his work has focused on the internal stimulus effects of drugs and the problem of drug dependence. He has published articles on the reinforcing, aversive and discriminative effects of drugs and on drug-produced changes in eating, drinking and loco-motor activity.

Foreword

In Western societies we are becoming increasingly aware of the impact of drugs in every-day life. Many of us use drugs such as nicotine and caffeine regularly and frequently. Some of us also use drugs as medicines or to cope with the pressures of life. Some people use 'social drugs' such as alcohol or marijuana to produce changes in the ways they feel, think or act. This book reviews research on the effects of the so-called psychoactive drugs, which can change our behaviour and our experience, in experimental, social and therapeutic settings.

Research in psychopharmacology has as its basic aim an understanding of the ways in which human behaviour is changed by drugs and an appreciation of the mechanisms through which such changes are brought about. Such knowledge may contribute to the development of new and better medicines for use in psychiatry and to the search for effective treatment for the problems which can arise when drugs are misused.

In order to achieve its aims, psychopharmacology is obliged to be eclectic in its approach to gathering relevant data. We have tried here to produce a book which reflects the diversity of psychopharmacology and which demonstrates the complexity and richness of this subject at present. The chapters have been written by experienced researchers and teachers drawn from the disciplines of psychology, pharmacology and psychiatry. The chapters range widely in their methodological orientation and in their contents. We hope that readers will be led thereby to appreciate how this diversity of expertise contributes to our knowledge about psychoactive substances. Increased knowledge will help us to cope more adequately with social problems of drug use and abuse and to recognize the potential and limitations of drug-based therapies for psychiatric illness.

D. J. Sanger
D. E. Blackman

1 Introduction to psychopharmacology and basic neuropharmacology

A. J. Greenshaw, D. J. Sanger *and* D. E. Blackman

Introduction

A willingness to take medicines seems to be one of the most funda-mental of human attributes. Of the enormous variety of drugs which doctors prescribe or which we prescribe for ourselves, many have effects on mood or experience. It seems that the use of such psycho-tropic drugs is ubiquitous. In all human societies past and present psychotropic drugs have been used avidly either in attempts to escape from unpleasant reality and achieve some transcendent or heavenly state or, alternatively, to return abnormal mental states to normality. Thus psychopharmacology, which in the most general meaning of the term refers to the study of the ways in which drugs alter psychological processes, has a long history and a broad scope. However, it has been only within recent decades that the investigation of psychotropic drug action has become an empirically based and sophisticated scientific discipline.

The purpose of this book is to provide the reader with a review of contemporary research in psychopharmacology. The essential aims of the discipline are to categorize the known substances which affect human mental processes and behaviour and to search for an understanding of the ways in which these drugs act. In addition to these basic scientific objectives psychopharmacology is also an important applied research area because, like other aspects of pharmacology, one of its aims is the discovery and development of more effective and safer medicines.

As the reader progresses through this book it will become clear that psychopharmacology is a diverse area of study involving aspects of psychology, pharmacology, chemistry, medicine and sociology. This very diversity, of course, makes psychopharmacology complex. It also makes it a rich and fascinating research area. In subsequent chapters of this book there will be descriptions of the ways in which psychotropic drugs are used clinically and non-clinically, accounts of changes in human and animal behaviour produced by drugs and attempts at explaining drug action both in psychological and biochemical terms. In the present chapter we present some general concepts which should aid the reader to deal with the more specialized material which follows. This chapter also contains some basic information on the ways in which drugs can affect the biochemistry of nerves.

Fundamentals of psychopharmacological research

Although we all feel we know what drugs are, the term drug is, in fact, extremely difficult to define with any precision. Broad definitions such as: 'any chemical agent which has an effect on living protoplasm' (Leavitt, 1974) seem to be too wide to be helpful scientifically; but attempts to provide narrower definitions would almost certainly not cover all the relevant possibilities. However, it seems rather less difficult to define the more circumscribed category of agents known as psychotropic drugs: a psychotropic (or psychoactive, which is a synonymous term) drug can be defined as a substance which, when taken, gives rise to changes in mental state or behaviour.

The basic design of an experimental study in psychopharmacology involves the administration of a measured amount of a psychotropic drug (a dose) and the accurate quantification of the resulting changes in behaviour. There are two basic approaches to such research. On the one hand behaviour can be used as a tool for studying different drugs, whereas, in contrast, it is also possible to use drugs as experimental tools for investigating psychological processes.

In the first approach, a well-understood aspect of behaviour is chosen and the ways in which this behaviour is altered by a variety of drugs investigated. Thus, to give a specific example, it is important for several reasons to discover how different drugs affect memory. The researcher interested in this problem would choose a test of memory which is quite thoroughly understood and then would measure the alterations in performance in this test produced by different drugs. Research of this type is described in Chapter 6.

The second general approach to research in psychopharmacology involves using drugs to learn more about behaviour. In this case, drugs are chosen for study whose mechanisms of action at either the behavioural or biochemical level are well known. These drugs can then be used to provide an understanding of basic psychological or biological aspects of particular behavioural phenomena. To provide one example, it is known that many drugs which are used with some success in treating mental depression produce changes in the activity of certain chemicals in the brain (Chapter 7). This finding has led to the development of theories concerning biochemical processes which may be correlated with depression and, more generally, to an improved knowledge of the brain mechanisms associated with mood.

Many other examples of the use of drugs as tools for the study of behaviour and, conversely, ways in which behaviour is utilized for the investigation of different drugs will be found throughout this book. As has been pointed out elsewhere (Sanger and Blackman, 1982), however, the distinction between these two approaches to research is not usually as clear as might be hoped. This is because there are few drugs whose pharmacological properties are known completely and few patterns of behaviour which psychologists would claim to understand thoroughly. Thus, much, perhaps most, research in psychopharmacology involves interactions between imperfectly understood pharmacological and psychological variables. Nevertheless, this research has given rise to rapid progress in our knowledge of both drugs and psychological processes.

The classification of psychotropic drugs

Classification and the organization of data are the corner-stone of most scientific activities. Within the relatively young science of psychopharmacology, classification is perhaps a little more difficult than in other scientific fields because of the wide range of levels of analysis with which psychopharmacologists are concerned, from molecular chemistry to integrated behaviour. The single factor around which psychopharmacology is focused is a concern with drugs, and the classification of psychotropic drugs might, at first sight, seem to be the simple key to the organization of the subject. However, psychotropic drugs may be classified in many ways with different categorizations reflecting the various levels of analysis ranging from a systematic analysis of chemical structures, through effects on the activity of isolated biological tissues, to a description of their effects on the behaviour of animals and men.

A broad and simple outline of the main classes of psychotropic drugs is presented in Table 1.1. This categorization relies heavily on the major effects which drugs exert on human psychological functions and includes both drugs used in medicine and drugs taken for non-clinical reasons either legally or illegally. Even this distinction between medical and non-medical use, however, cuts across these categories as there are some drugs with important clinical uses which are also subject to misuse.

The first two categories listed in Table 1.1, neuroleptics and antidepressants, contain drugs which are used by psychiatrists in treating the serious mental disorders of schizophrenia and depression. Although it would not be suggested that such drugs cure psychoses, it is generally believed that they are effective in treating many symptoms of schizophrenia and depression and go some way towards normalizing the grossly abnormal cognitive states experienced by people suffering from these disorders. Anxiolytics are also drugs which are thought to have beneficial effects in treating psychological disorders, in this case severe anxiety. However, the most widely used anxiolytic drugs, the benzodiazepines, seem also to be subject to some misuse (Petursson and Lader, 1981) while neuroleptic and antidepressant agents seem to have no potential for abuse. In addition to their use in the treatment of anxiety some benzodiazepines are used for inducing sleep. Barbiturates have also had considerable use as sedatives but have greater potential toxicity and are more likely to give rise to dependence and abuse than are benzodiazepines.

Some analgesic drugs are also correctly classed as psychotropic agents. In particular, the opium derivatives including morphine, heroin and codeine, which are powerful painkillers and thus important medical tools, also have other effects on behaviour. These include the production of a euphoric state which may be an important reason why some opiate drugs have been widely abused.

Table 1.1   Classes of psychotropic drugs

Class	Major effects and medical uses	Selected examples
Neuroleptics (major tranquillizers)	Treatment of schizophrenic symptoms	Chlorpromazine Pimozide Haloperidol
Antidepressants	Treatment of mental depression	Imipramine Mianserin
Anxiolytics (minor tranquillizers)	Alleviation of anxiety	Benzodiazepines such as Diazepam
Sedatives/hypnotics	Induction of sleep	Barbiturates Benzodiazepines
Analgesics	Alleviation of pain	Opiates such as Morphine
Cognition activators	Improvement in cognitive abilities	Piracetam Vasopressin
Anorectics	Reductions in hunger and food intake	Fenfluramine Amphetamine
Psychomotor stimulants	Increase in activity, improvement in mood	Amphetamine Cocaine, Caffeine, Nicotine
Psychedelics	Distortion of perception (alteration in sensory processes)	LSD Mescaline Cannabis

Another category of drugs which may have important medical uses includes those which we have referred to as activators of cognition. These are drugs which can improve mental functions such as attention and memory. For many years psychopharmacologists and laymen have been fascinated by the prospect of a 'memory drug' but research has met with little success. Recent research, however, has had the more realistic aim of searching for agents which improve cognitive abilities in patients suffering from disorders such as dementia without necessarily expecting such drugs to improve normal mental abilities. Modern research has made steady progress and a number of drugs have been claimed to exert cognitive activating properties.

With the exception of anorectic agents which are used to reduce appetite to aid the treatment of obesity, the remaining drug categories shown in Table 1.1 contain substances which have few, if any, medical uses. Nevertheless, these drugs have a variety of profound effects on behaviour which have led to their widespread non-clinical use.

Stimulants, such as amphetamine and cocaine, increase activity levels and can give rise to a heightened sense of well-being and perhaps an unrealistic level of cheerfulness. In general, however, they seem not to be effective at alleviating depression. Such drugs have also had some popularity with some athletes in illicit attempts to improve sporting performance (Laties and Weiss, 1981). The much milder stimulant drugs, caffeine and nicotine, are, of course, very widely used presumably for their psychotropic actions. With the probable exception of alcohol, caffeine is the world's most widely taken psychotropic drug as it, or one of its derivates, is contained in coffee, tea and a variety of other drinks and foods.

The psychedelic drugs are substances whose major effects are to produce changes in sensory and perceptual processes. Drugs such as LSD and mescaline give rise to very profound alterations in visual perception and these actions have led to their being called hallucinogenic drugs. It seems, however, that these drugs do not produce true hallucinations in the sense that the drug taker believes in the existence of his or her drug-induced perceptions. Cannabis can also be classed as a minor psychedelic drug as it appears to produce minor changes in perception as well as changes in mood and in cognitive processes such as memory.

The actions of drugs on brain chemistry

Associated with all cognitive states and patterns of behaviour are changes in the biochemical activity of the brain although it may not always be entirely necessary for us to understand these changes in order to develop an adequate understanding of behaviour as such. Psychotropic drugs can, however, be assumed to act directly on the chemical activity of the brain to give rise to changes in behaviour. A complete understanding of the actions of psychotropic drugs, therefore, will almost certainly require an integration of both psychological and physiological or biochemical knowledge.

Psychologists interested in the effects of drugs are often criticized, quite correctly, for knowing too little about the biochemistry and general pharmacology of drug action. On the other hand, pharmacologists could occasionally benefit from a deeper understanding of psychological concepts. The present book is aimed primarily at those interested in psychological aspects of psychopharmacology. However, in order adequately to appreciate much of the information contained in subsequent chapters a basic knowledge of neuropharmacology (i.e. the effects of drugs on the activity of nerves) will be helpful. The remaining sections of this chapter, therefore, present some information about the ways in which drugs can alter biochemical processes in the central nervous system.

Principles of neural transmission

Activity in the mammalian central nervous system may be envisaged in terms of two basic processes. Within a nerve cell, or neuron, activity takes the form of electrical impulses, or action potentials. These are transmitted along the length of the neuron, the axon, to terminal regions distal to the cell body. The resultant excitation of these terminal regions causes the release of chemical activators called neurotransmitters into special junctional regions between nerve cells. These junctions are called synapses. Neurotransmitters released into these junctional regions, or synaptic clefts, may interact reversibly with specialized parts of the postsynaptic membrane that act as receptors. The interaction of neurotransmitter molecules with these receptors results in a change in the state of excitation of the neurons. Such changes in excitation may be facilitatory, giving rise to action potentials in these neurons, with a consequent release of neurotransmitters further down the line. Alternatively, activity in certain neurons may have inhibitory effects on others, with a resultant attenuation of ongoing activity or a damping of the effects of other, excitatory, inputs. An excellent and detailed exposition of neurotransmission at the biophysical level has been compiled by Katz (1966).

There are a number of substances in the central nervous system that are fairly well established as neurotransmitters: acetylcholine (ACh); noradrenaline (NA); dopamine (DA); 5-hydroxytryptamine (5HT); gamma aminobutyric acid (GABA); glycine (Gly).

In recent years interest has focused on a number of additional molecules, both peptides and amines, as possible mediators of neural regulation. Endogenous neuropeptides such as enkephalins, endorphins and substance P have recently received immense attention (see Iversen and Iversen, 1981, p. 69), although it is unclear in most cases whether they act as neurotransmitters or have some other less well defined function in neural transmission.

The processes by which neurons communicate with each other are of course more complex than any outline of bioelectrical wiring and neurochemical switching might suggest. It was first thought that each neuron contained a single neurotransmitter (Dale, 1935), i.e. DA, 5HT, GABA or one of the other substances listed above. However, this tenet, known as 'Dale's principle', is not strictly correct as it is now established that neurotransmitters may coexist in certain neurons. This observation, together with the growing variety of compounds that may be involved in neural regulation, indicates the complexity of the processes involved. The present discussion cannot provide a detailed view of this area. However, current controversies have recently been extensively reviewed in an article and accompanying commentary that, although demanding, indicates the excitement of this field (Dismukes, 1979).

The pharmacology of synaptic activity

Many psychoactive drugs exert their effects at the synaptic level and it is therefore appropriate to consider some of the fundamental features of brain chemistry here. For our purposes synaptic activity may be envisaged in terms of several component functions illustrated schematically in Figure 1.1.

The main features of neuronal regulation processes are:

(1) Transport along the axon of substances involved in neuronal metabolism and in the synthesis of neuroactive compounds (e.g. neurotransmitters).
(2) Synthesis of neuroactive compounds.
(3) Storage of neuroactive compounds within the presynaptic terminal region.
(4) The release of neurotransmitters through the presynaptic cell membrane into the synaptic cleft.
(5) The activation of specific receptors on the neural membrane by neurotransmitters in the synaptic cleft.
(6) The uptake of neurotransmitters or their constituents from the synaptic cleft into presynaptic terminal regions.
(7) The breakdown, or catabolism, of neuroactive compounds either in the synaptic cleft or in the presynaptic terminal region.

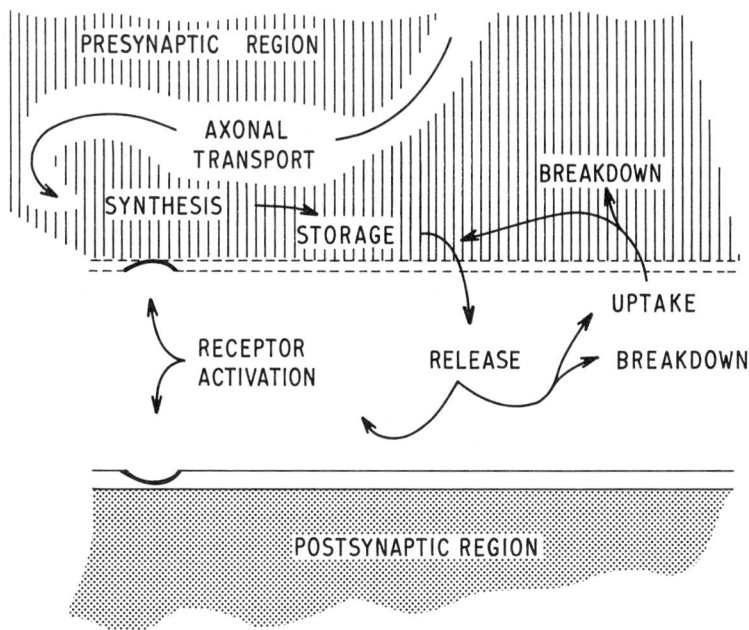

Fig. 1.1   A schematic representation of the basic features of neural pharmacology. The shaded area represents the presynaptic terminal region of one neuron. The postsynaptic region of a neighbouring neuron is represented by the dotted area. The unshaded area between them represents the synaptic cleft. This figure illustrates the general localization of different dynamic aspects of synaptic activity.

In Figure 1.1 receptor activation is shown at both the presynaptic and postsynaptic membranes. Whereas postsynaptic membrane receptors are usually related to communication between different neurons, the existence of presynaptic or auto-receptors is indicative of one of the numerous feedback mechanisms that serve to regulate neural processes. In certain neurons, the quantity of neurotransmitters released into the synaptic cleft may be regulated by the activation of these auto-receptors. The availability of transmitter substances in the presynaptic region also serves to regulate the rate of synthesis of these compounds and their mechanisms of storage in nerve cells.

Synthesis and metabolism of major neurotransmitters

The following pages (pp. 10–19) contain detailed biochemical material which will be useful in understanding the rest of this book.

Readers who are unfamiliar with this material may wish to use it for reference purposes rather than read it straight through at this stage.

An appreciation of the biochemical pathways involved in the synthesis and metabolism of neurotransmitters is crucial for an understanding of the ways in which drugs may selectively alter neural activity. The best understood pathways are those involving acetylcholine (ACh) and the monoamines noradrenaline (NA), dopamine (DA) and 5-hydroxytryptamine (5HT). The catecholamines NA and DA are intimately related in that they share a common synthetic pathway, whereas ACh and the indoleamine 5HT must be considered separately. The basic layout of each of these pathways is presented in Figure 1.2 for the catecholamines and Figures 1.3 and 1.4 for 5HT and ACh.

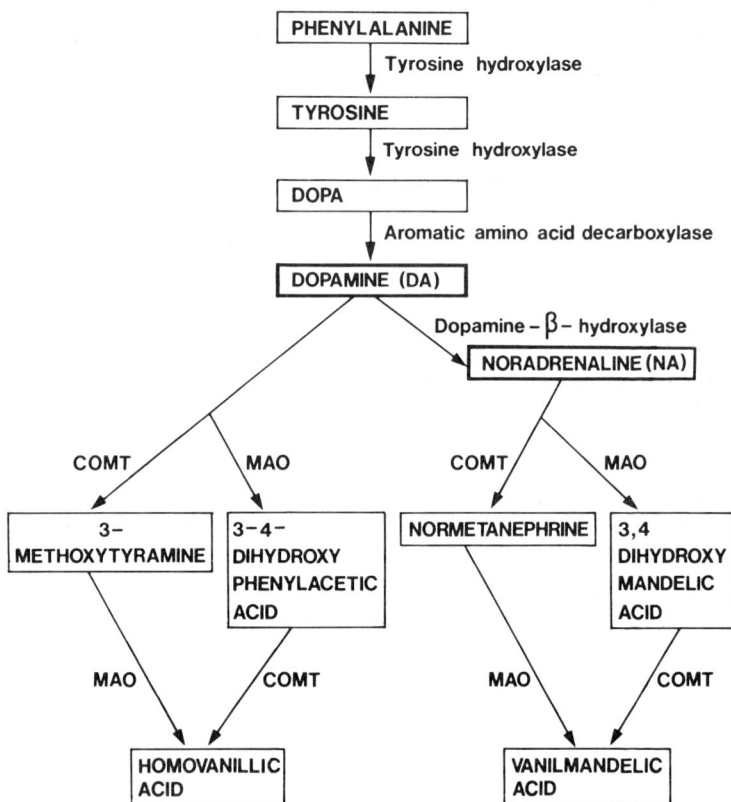

Fig. 1.2   The synthesis and metabolism of noradrenaline and dopamine (MAO is monoamine oxidase and COMT is catechol-o-methyltransferase).

In the case of the catecholamines, both NA and DA are synthe-
sized from a common precursor, phenylalanine (an amino acid obtained from food), which is converted through tyrosine to dopa by
hydroxylation reactions which are mediated by the enzyme tyrosine
hydroxylase. Dopa is then converted to DA by decarboxylation involving another enzyme, aromatic amino acid decarboxylase; also
known as dopa decarboxylase. In noradrenergic nerve terminals DA
is then further converted to NA through another hydroxylation
reaction involving the enzyme dopamine-β-hydroxylase. DA and NA
are broken down by a further two enzymes, monoamine oxidase
(MAO) and catechol-o-methyltransferase (COMT), to form their respective metabolites, homovanillic acid (HVA) and vanilmandelic
acid (VMA).

The synthesis of 5HT from the precursor tryptophan similarly
involves hydroxylation and decarboxylation reactions (Figure 1.3). In
this case it is of interest that the precursor tryptophan may be converted,

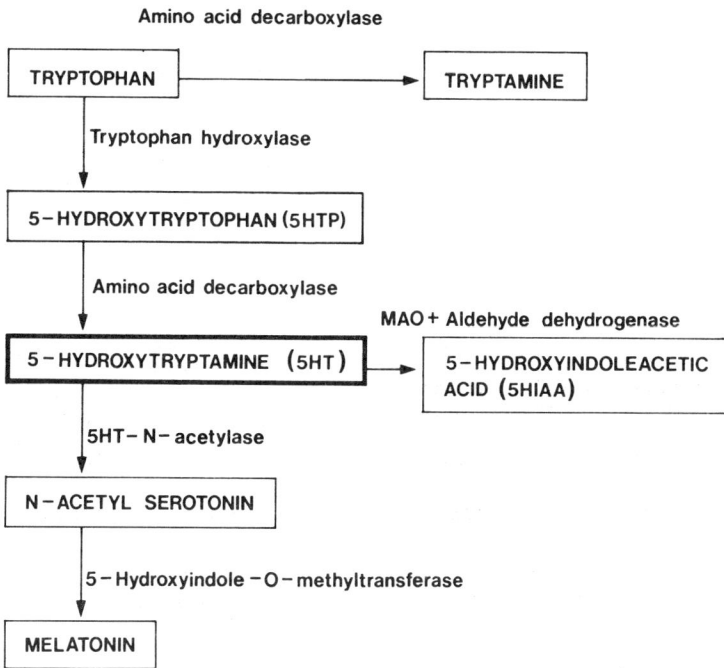

Fig. 1.3   The synthesis and metabolism of 5-hydroxytryptamine (5HT).

via a decarboxylation step, to tryptamine, a compound that may also be involved in neural regulation processes (Boulton and Juorio, 1982). 5HT is broken down through its conversion to 5-hydroxyindoleacetic acid (5HIAA), or through the formation of N-acetyl serotonin to melatonin. The various enzymes involved in these reactions are shown in Figure 1.3.

The monoamine neurotransmitters (DA, NA and 5HT) may be converted to their respective metabolites either in the synaptic cleft or in the presynaptic terminal region. There are uptake systems in the presynaptic membranes of monoaminergic neurons that readily transfer transmitter molecules from the synaptic cleft back into the terminal areas. Here monoamines are either replaced in storage or are broken down into their respective metabolites by MAO.

In cholinergic neuronal systems ACh is mainly broken down in the

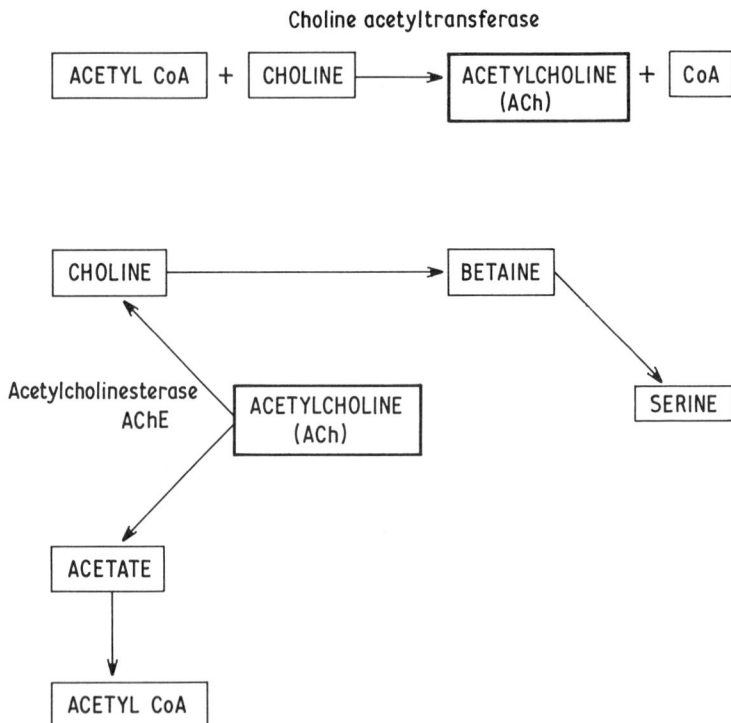

Choline acetyltransferase

ACETYL CoA + CHOLINE ⟶ ACETYLCHOLINE (ACh) + CoA

CHOLINE ⟶ BETAINE

Acetylcholinesterase AChE

ACETYLCHOLINE (ACh)

BETAINE ⟶ SERINE

ACETATE

ACETYL CoA

Fig. 1.4   The synthesis and metabolism of acetylcholine (ACh). (AChE is acetylcholinesterase.)

synaptic cleft into its constituents choline and acetate (see Figure 1.4). In these neurons the presynaptic membrane has an uptake system for choline. This system may also transport ACh, but the extremely rapid breakdown of this molecule by acetylcholinesterase (AChE) minimizes ACh uptake. The formation of ACh in the presynaptic region is governed by the enzyme acetyltransferase, although the main factor limiting this process is the availability of the precursor choline. These reactions are also illustrated schematically in Figure 1.4.

Multiple receptor types and receptor-binding

Our understanding of the effects of drugs at the synaptic level comes largely from the use of specific biochemical and electrophysiological techniques involving both isolated tissue preparations (*in vitro* procedures) and the use of whole animals (*in vivo* procedures). It would be inappropriate to describe these methods here as detailed information is readily available elsewhere (Iversen *et al.*, 1975) and this material is generally beyond the scope of the present discussion. However, one particular issue, that of receptor binding, is important enough to deserve some consideration.

As outlined earlier, neurotransmitters exert their effects by interacting with specific receptors situated on postsynaptic (and, in certain cases, presynaptic) membranes. Just as there may often be more than one type of neurotransmitter involved in the activity of a single neuron, there may also be different types of receptors. Furthermore, a single neurotransmitter may exert its actions on different types of receptors that interact specifically with that transmitter. Unfortunately the issue is every bit as complex as it sounds. Not surprisingly there are many controversies in contemporary receptor pharmacology. For certain transmitters it appears to be well established that multiple receptor types exist. For example, it is generally accepted that acetylcholine interacts with two types of receptor called muscarinic and nicotinic receptors respectively. Noradrenaline interacts with both α (Type 1 and 2) and β (Type 1 and 2) receptors; and dopamine appears to bind to at least two (D_1 and D_2) and possibly four receptors (see Creese, 1982 for an attempt at a current synthesis). If we were to extend the list to various other possible receptors for neuroactive compounds it would be very long indeed. Also, this is a fast-moving field and some recently discovered receptors have important implications in the study of behavioural effects of drugs, e.g. the respective NA and DA auto-receptors α_2 and D_2

The current increase in postulated receptor types is attributable to recent advances in the field of 'receptor-binding' (Snyder and Bennett, 1976). Receptor-binding techniques involve the labelling of receptors with specific radioactive ligands (i.e. substances that bind to receptors). These procedures allow pharmacologists to identify different types of receptors and to determine their quantitative distribution in different types of tissue or in different areas of the brain. Such techniques are proving to be increasingly useful in determining the relative specificity of different drugs in terms of their actions at different classes of receptors.

Drug-induced modulation of neural activity

Effects of drugs on neuronal activity are commonly visualized in terms of the various components of neural activity shown in Figure 1.1.

At the receptor level drugs may exert excitatory effects at receptor sites and thus be described as agonists. Alternatively, they may act as antagonists by competitively blocking receptors, thus making them unresponsive to endogenous agonists (i.e. transmitters) or their exogenous analogues. Exogenously applied agonists, therefore, tend to mimic the effects of increased availability of neurotransmitter molecules, whereas antagonists will have opposite effects. Certain compounds may paradoxically exhibit both properties, and are thus mixed agonist/antagonists.

Uptake blockers (e.g. cocaine) act by inhibiting uptake mechanisms in presynaptic membranes, thereby increasing the availability of transmitters at receptor sites. Agents that facilitate transmitter release such as amphetamine similarly have the effect of facilitating transmitter activity. Conversely, enzymes involved in the synthesis of neurotransmitters can be inhibited by drugs such as the tyrosine hydroxylase inhibitor α-methyl-p-tyrosine (AMPT). Alternatively, transmitter stores can be depleted by compounds such as reserpine. Both types of drug will, therefore, inhibit neuronal activity.

Typically, psychoactive drugs may act by affecting a number of the processes outlined in Figure 1.1 and specificity of action is often a contentious issue. For example, the psychomotor stimulant drug amphetamine blocks the uptake of NA from the synaptic cleft, causes a release of monoamines from storage vesicles into the synapse and is a weak MAO inhibitor. Another example of non-specificity of action may be seen in the effects of a compound with functionally opposite effects. Chlorpromazine, a neuroleptic drug, acts by blocking NA, DA and 5HT receptors. In this case, although the major influence of this drug is on catecholamine receptors, the effects of chlorpromazine on 5HT receptors seriously limit its usefulness as a research tool for manipulating catecholamine activity. The lack of absolute specificity of drug effects makes the task of identifying neuropharmacological mechanisms of drug-induced behavioural changes or of clinical activity a difficult one. Nevertheless, it is possible to choose drugs on the basis of their relative specificity of action for the purpose of manipulating various aspects of neural activity. In order to illustrate this possibility clearly, it may be useful to consider the various manipulations that can be carried out with respect to one neurotransmitter − in this case NA.

Noradrenergic activity can most directly be increased with the application of different noradrenergic agonists. For this purpose compounds such as isoprenaline and phenylephrine may be used. Isoprenaline acts mainly at β-noradrenergic receptors whereas phenylephrine tends to activate α-noradrenergic receptors. A less direct but similar effect may be obtained by administering precursors of neurotransmitters; in this case with a compound such as phenylalanine or l-dopa. Similar effects may be achieved with the use of compounds that facilitate the release of NA through the presynaptic membrane. Amphetamine is one such drug, although, as described earlier, it has other effects at the synaptic level. Blockade of uptake mechanisms with compounds such as desmethylimipramine will also facilitate NA activity. Inhibiting the activity of the enzymes MAO or COMT will result in a decrease in the breakdown of NA although this manipulation will obviously have similar effects on the other monoamines (see Figure 1.3). Pargyline is a commonly used MAO inhibitor and tropolane is an effective inhibitor of COMT. The result of any of the last three treatments will be an increased availability of NA in the synaptic cleft. A combination of these effects, e.g. uptake-blockade and inhibition of catabolism, by the administration of two drugs, e.g. pargyline and desmethylimipramine, will be more effective than either treatment alone. In this regard it is easy to see how a drug like amphetamine can exert such marked effects on behaviour for it acts on uptake and release mechanisms and on MAO activity.

Conversely, noradrenergic activity may be attenuated by a number

Table 1.2 A classification of some of the more commonly used compounds in relation to their effects on the pharmacology of synaptic activity

Transmitter	NA	DA	5HT	ACh
Precursors	Phenylalanine Tyrosine Dopa	Phenylalanine Tyrosine Dopa	Tryptophan 5-Hydroxytryptophan	Choline
Synthesis inhibitors	AMPT FLA-63 Disulfiram	AMPT	p-Chlorophenylalanine p-Chloroamphetamine	—
Depleters	Reserpine Tetrabenazine	Reserpine Tetrabenazine	Reserpine	Hemicholinium (Depletion is secondary to blockade of the uptake of choline)
Uptake blockers	Amphetamine Cocaine	Amphetamine Cocaine Benztropine	Cocaine Zimelidine Fluoxetine Fenfluramine	Hemicholinium
Inhibitors of catabolism	MAO inhibitors (Pargyline) COMT inhibitors (Tropolane)	MAO inhibitors (Pargyline) COMT inhibitors (Tropolane)	MAO inhibitors (Pargyline)	Neostigmine Physostigmine

Agonists	(α) Clonidine Phenylephrine (β) Isoprenaline	Apomorphine Piribedil	Quipazine Bufotenin 5-Methoxytryptamine	(Nicotinic) Nicotine Carbachol (Muscarinic) Muscarine Oxotremorine
Antagonists	(α) Phenoxybenzamine Phentolamine (β) Propranolol	Pimozide Haloperidol α-Flupenthixol	Methysergide Metergoline Cyproheptadine	(Nicotinic) Mecamylamine Hexamethonium (Muscarinic) Atropine Scopolamine
Neurotoxins	DSP4 6-OHDA	6-OHDA	5,6-DHT 5,7-DHT	—

of pharmacological manipulations. The most direct of these is through the administration of antagonists that competitively block NA receptors. Phentolamine is a fairly specific antagonist at α noradrenergic receptors and propranolol similarly acts as a blocker of β receptors. Inhibition of NA synthesis with compounds such as the dopamine β-hydroxylase inhibitor diethyldithiocarbamate (DDC), also known as disulfiram, will decrease the availability of NA in the synaptic cleft. Here, it is of interest to consider the possible alternatives in choosing synthesis inhibitors. DDC will reduce the synthesis of NA without affecting the availability of DA, whereas a compound such as AMPT will reduce the synthesis at both DA and NA (see Figure 1.2). This is a good example of how differential manipulations of neurochemicals with common biosynthetic pathways can be achieved. Clearly there are various possibilities of this sort, particularly in relation to the production of active metabolites of the major transmitters.

There is, then, a wide range of available compounds that may be used as research tools to alter synaptic activity in relation to different neurotransmitters. A guide to some of the more commonly used drugs is presented in Table 1.2. Here drugs are arranged in order of their effects on different features of neural pharmacology for NA, DA, 5HT and ACh respectively.

In determining the suitability of various drugs for different experimental manipulations a number of factors have to be considered. Certain compounds are readily absorbed from the periphery into the central nervous system through the blood-brain barrier, others are not. This is an important feature of drug activity that precludes the use of certain compounds when drugs are to be administered peripherally. However, with specialized administration procedures, pharmacological substances may be delivered directly into the central nervous system, thereby avoiding this problem. Duration of action and reversibility of pharmacological effects must also be taken into account. Some experimental procedures involve repeated testing and these factors are of paramount importance under these circumstances. These considerations are a clear reflection of the necessary concern that all psychopharmacologists must have for purely pharmacological and biochemical aspects of drug activity.

No account of the influences of drugs on brain chemistry would be complete without some mention of our understanding of how different transmitter systems are arranged neuroanatomically. As a result of the pioneering histochemical work of Falck *et al.* (1962), the actual visualization of 'chemical pathways' in the central nervous system was achieved with histofluorescence techniques. This early work has led to a fairly detailed mapping of pathways for DA, NA and 5HT, although other neurochemical systems are not well established in this sense (Iversen *et al.*, 1978).

The elucidation of such neurochemical pathways has led to great advances in the analysis of neuropharmacological systems and behavioural change. This is particularly true for the catecholamine systems (Iversen, 1978). The measurement of behavioural change in relation to the manipulation of neural activity, particularly in discrete brain areas, is a rapidly expanding field. The issues are extremely complex and progress, while rapid in some specific areas, is generally slow. This is primarily due to the increasing number of substances that may be involved in the neural regulation of behaviour, together with our increasingly complex views of the neurochemical effects of drugs. Nevertheless, the potential of this research for an understanding of the ways in which pharmacological activity changes behaviour is tremendous.

This completes our short review of the basic principles of neuropharmacology. It can be seen that neuropharmacology can be a dauntingly complex field of study, and it is one in which great advances are currently being made. It is not our intention here to overwhelm the reader with details and complexities. However, as we have argued, a very basic knowledge of the principles of neuropharmacology may be advantageous in psychopharmacology, and with respect to subsequent chapters in this book. These chapters focus more directly on the effects of drugs on psychological rather than biochemical processes. Perhaps the present review may provide the reader who is unfamiliar with pharmacology with a useful taxonomy of the drugs whose behavioural effects are discussed in these chapters.

References

Boulton, A. A. and Juorio, A. V. (1982) Brain trace amines. In A. Lajtha (ed.) *Handbook of Neurochemistry*. Vol. 1. New York: Plenum Press, pp. 189–222.

Creese, I. (1982) Dopamine receptors explained. *Trends in Neuroscience 5*: 40–3.

Dale, H. H. (1935) Pharmacology and nerve endings. *Proceedings of the Royal Society of Medicine 28*: 319–32.

Dismukes, R. K. (1979) New concepts of molecular communication among neurons. *The Behavioural and Brain Sciences 2*: 409–48.

Falck, B., Hillarp, N. A., Thieme, G. and Tarp, A. (1962) Fluorescence of catecholamines and related compounds condensed with formaldehyde. *Journal of Histochemistry and Cytochemistry 10*: 348–54.

Iversen, L. L., Iversen, S. D. and Snyder, S. H. (eds) (1975) Biochemical principles and techniques in neuropharmacology. *Handbook of Psychopharmacology*. Vol. 1. New York: Plenum Press.

Iversen, L. L., Iversen, S. D. and Snyder, S. H. (eds) (1978) Chemical pathways in the brain. *Handbook of Psychopharmacology*. Vol. 9. New York: Plenum Press.

Iversen, S. D. (1978) Brain dopamine systems and behavior. In L. L. Iversen, S. D. Iversen and S. H. Snyder (eds) *Handbook of Psychopharmacology*. Vol. 8. New York: Plenum Press, pp. 333–84.

Iversen, S. D. and Iversen, L. L. (1981) *Behavioral Pharmacology* (2nd edn). New York: Oxford University Press.

Katz, B. (1966) *Nerve, Muscle and Synapse*. New York: McGraw Hill.

Laties, V. G. and Weiss, B. (1981) The amphetamine margin in sports. *Federation Proceedings 40*: 2689–92.

Leavitt, F. (1974) *Drugs and Behavior*. Philadelphia: W. B. Saunders.

Petursson, H. and Lader, M. H. (1981) Benzodiazepine dependence. *British Journal of Addiction 76*: 133–45.

Sanger, D. J. and Blackman, D. E. (1982) Drug-induced cognitive and behavioural change. In A. Burton (ed.) *The Pathology and Psychology of Cognition*. London: Methuen.

Snyder, S. H. and Bennett, J. P. (1976) Neurotransmitter receptors in the brain: biochemical identification. *Annual Review of Physiology 38*: 153–75.

2 Behavioural principles in psychopharmacology

James E. Barrett

Introduction

Although the effects of psychoactive drugs can be studied at many different levels, ultimately any analysis must address issues of a behavioural nature. Experiments involving isolated neurons or receptor activity, for example, take on added significance when related to the intact behaving organism. On a different level, psychiatric disorders are most clearly manifested and described as disturbances in behaviour. Drugs with potential therapeutic efficacy in psychiatry are clinically evaluated by their ability to alter the dominant behavioural symptoms of a particular disease. The excessive use of abused drugs is also characterized by marked changes in drug-taking and drug-induced behaviour. The conspicuousness and importance of behaviour under such conditions should not be interpreted as only indicating that it is merely a passive transmitter of changes or influences occurring at a different level. Often, as we shall see, behaviour itself and the variables that control it can play a prominent and active role in directly determining drug action.

The broad field of psychopharmacology embraces diverse disciplines that address issues which are eventually translated into questions about behaviour. Behavioural pharmacology, a field which combines principles taken from the experimental analysis of behaviour and experimental pharmacology, is an essential component of psychopharmacological research. An organism's behaviour is dynamically related to the environment in which that behaviour takes place. Interactions between behaviour and the environment not only alter behaviour but can also profoundly affect drug action. Research in behavioural pharmacology is designed, to a large extent, to reveal and understand behavioural and environmental mechanisms responsible for the actions of drugs on behaviour.

This chapter will first review some of the principles involved in the experimental study of behaviour and will then describe how these behavioural principles influence drug action. For the most part, the discussion will deal with research conducted with non-human animals. Aspects of drugs and human behaviour are treated more extensively in later sections of this book. It should be clear, however, that principles described in this chapter are of widespread importance and fundamental significance for an understanding of drug effects on behaviour.

The observation and experimental analysis of behaviour

As has been the case with other developing fields, the experimental study of behaviour initially confronted a number of philosophical and methodological issues. Much of the original controversy has abated in recent years and substantial progress has now been made in understanding and accepting the fact that behaviour can be objectively and experimentally investigated. Cumulative advances in the analysis of behaviour have provided techniques which permit the development and maintenance of a wide variety of behaviours that are remarkably stable over time, manipulable over a wide range, reproducible within and across species, and sensitive to a number of interventions. The successful use of these procedures in behavioural pharmacology has had the dual advantage of broadening our understanding of both behaviour and principles of drug action. This chapter will be concerned primarily with providing a general description of some of the basic procedures used in the behavioural pharmacology laboratory. We will then examine how the effects of various drugs are determined by behavioural variables.

For the most part, research studying the effects of drugs on behaviour has been conducted with two basic types of procedures. One procedure utilizes *unconditioned* behaviour. In some cases, uncon-ditioned behaviour is simply monitored or measured, as with locomotor activity. Under other conditions, unconditioned behaviour is produced or *elicited* by presenting specific stimuli and is then brought under experimental control by arranging that the response occur to stimuli other than those originally responsible for its occurrence. For example, Pavlov (1927) performed extensive studies using the unconditioned salivary response to food and to stimuli paired with food. This type of procedure has been termed classical or *respondent conditioning*.

The second procedure, termed *operant conditioning*, uses the tech-niques and methods developed by Skinner (1938) to investigate behaviour controlled by its consequences. A vast amount of work in behavioural pharmacology has been conducted using these operant conditioning methods and this topic is discussed in greater detail below. Extensive treatment of principles of behavioural analysis, conditioning and learning can be found in several texts (e.g. Black-man, 1974).

Unconditioned and respondent behaviour

Unconditioned behaviour involves those activities of the organism that require no specific training or conditioning process. Such behav-iours are usually part of the normal behavioural repertoire of a species and are, therefore, 'spontaneous' or naturally occurring in suitable environments (e.g. locomotor activity, food or water intake or sexual behaviour). Although factors responsible for the occurrence of these behaviours presumably lie in the organism's distant evolutionary and biological past, certain unconditioned responses can also be brought under more direct and immediate experimental control through the procedures first discovered and systematically explored by Pavlov (1927). These procedures essentially consist of expanding the range of stimuli capable of producing or eliciting a response. In respondent conditioning, previously non-effective (conditional) stimuli acquire the ability to produce or *elicit* a response by virtue of their temporal association with an unconditional stimulus (e.g. food) which is capable of eliciting a response without prior conditioning. Thus, when a distinctive noise, such as a tone, is repeatedly presented at the same time as or shortly before food is given, the tone acquires the ability to *elicit* many of the same responses originally limited only to food.

Respondent behaviours depend primarily on *antecedent* events or stimuli that elicit particular responses. Typically, respondent behaviours do not undergo progressive differentiation in that the response to a stimulus paired with food is similar in many respects to that occurring when food is presented. Respondent conditioning procedures, then, do not establish *new* responses. Instead, after conditioning, the same response, or one very similar, simply occurs to an expanded range of stimuli.

A later section will briefly discuss drug effects on respondent behaviour although, relative to research using operant conditioning procedures, there has been little work examining the effects of drugs on such behaviour.

The effects of drugs on unconditioned behaviour such as locomotor activity or drug-induced stereotyped movements have been studied more extensively. Thus, many researchers have made use of measures of locomotor activity in novel or familiar environments or of the intake of food and water for studying drug action (Baez, 1976; Robbins, 1977). Several types of social behaviour including aggression and sexual activity have also been investigated in pharmacological experiments (Miczek and Barry, 1976). Many investigations of drug effects on unconditioned behaviour have as their purpose the analysis of drug action at the pharmacological and biochemical levels and we therefore have considerable knowledge of the neurochemical mechanisms in the central nervous system which are modified during drug-induced changes in, for example, feeding and drinking. The present chapter, in contrast, is primarily concerned with statements of principle which relate the actions of drugs to behavioural and environmental factors. It is in this area that the study of operant behaviour has made the most significant contribution to psychopharmacology.

Operant behaviour

In contrast to respondent behaviour, operant behaviour is controlled by *consequent* rather than antecedent events. Operant behaviour is established, maintained and further modified by its consequences. Although respondent behaviours are more or less reflexively elicited by specific stimuli, operant behaviours are said to be *emitted* in the absence of any identifiable eliciting stimuli; depending on the consequences, operant behaviours are either more or less likely to be repeated in the future.

Operant behaviours occur for reasons not always specifiable. They may have some initially low probability of occurrence or they may never have occurred previously. Novel operant responses can be established by the technique of 'shaping' or successive approximation. In the process of shaping, behaviours which resemble or approximate some final desired form are selected, increased in frequency and further differentiated by the provision of a suitable consequence. For example, lever pressing in an experimentally naïve, food-deprived rat can be conditioned by the delivery of food following responses that initially only roughly approximate a lever press. However, as the consequent food increases responses that immediately precede its presentation, behaviour progressively changes to more closely approximate the final lever-pressing response. Often, the final features of a behaviour that has been differentially shaped may bear little or no resemblance to its initial form. Behaviour that has evolved under such contingencies can be understood only by examining the individual's history. Although some behaviours appear completely novel or unique, it is likely that the final product emerged as a continuous process directly related to earlier forms. In short, operant conditioning, unlike respondent conditioning, can establish new responses. The manner in which these responses are then maintained and further modified by their consequences has been the subject of extensive study and has had tremendous impact on the development of operant behavioural pharmacology.

In principle, it is possible to separate operant and respondent behaviour in a number of ways; in practice, however, rigorous distinctions between these behaviours are often quite difficult. Under some conditions, the processes of operant and respondent conditioning occur concurrently and blend together, almost indistinguishably. Under other conditions, elicited responses can also be modified and eventually maintained, often by the same stimuli, when those stimuli occur as a consequence of responding. This blending of operant and respondent behaviour may be more common than is generally acknowledged. The primary distinctions between operant and respondent behaviours now appear to be the way these behaviours are produced and the possible differential susceptibility to modification by consequent events. Respondent behaviour is produced by the presentation of eliciting stimuli; characteristic features of these behaviours are rather easily changed by altering the features of the eliciting stimulus such as its intensity, duration or frequency of presentation. Under all these conditions, however, the response remains essentially the same.

Operant behaviour depends to a large extent on its consequences. Complex behaviour can develop from quite simple relationships. When current behaviour is seen as an instance of the organism's previous history acting together with more immediate consequences, one gains a greater appreciation for the continuity of behaviour in time (Morse, 1966). Current behaviour is often exceedingly difficult to understand because many prior influences or consequences have ceased to operate. However, the residual behavioural effects of these influences are probably still present. The effects of a particular consequence can be quite different depending on the behaviour that exists at the time that the event occurs. An individual's prior history, then, is important not only because it has shaped present behaviour, but also because it will undoubtedly determine the specific ways in which that individual responds to the current environment. As we will see, prior behavioural experience can have a marked effect in determining how a drug will change behaviour.

Processes of reinforcement and punishment   Two key principles in operant behaviour and in behavioural pharmacology have been *reinforcement* and *punishment*. Reinforcement is a process in which an *increase* in responding occurs following the presentation or termination of some event. Punishment is a process in which the presentation or withdrawal of an event following a response produces a *decrease* in subsequent responding. It is important to note that reinforcement and punishment are descriptive, empirical processes that refer to relationships between behaviour and its consequences rather than explanatory terms. The defining characteristics of reinforcers and punishers depend on how behaviour is changed, not on the characteristics of the events themselves. An event presented under one condition may function as a reinforcer, whereas under a different condition that same event may function as a punisher. The behavioural effects of most environmental events are not fixed but can depend on many factors such as prior experience, features of ongoing behaviour and other conditions existing at the time that that event occurs.

Schedules of reinforcement   One of the important factors in determining whether an event will be reinforcing or punishing is the way that the event is and has been scheduled with regard to behaviour. Many features of operant behaviour, including its frequency of occurrence, idiosyncratic form and susceptibility to further modification, depend on the consequences of past behaviour acting together with current environmental conditions. The study of operant conditioning has focused on extensive analyses of these conditions using *schedules of reinforcement* (Ferster and Skinner, 1957).

A schedule of reinforcement is, by definition, a 'prescription for initiating and terminating stimuli, either discriminative or reinforcing, in time and in relation to responses' (Morse, 1966, p. 56). Our previous discussion of shaping, reinforcement and punishment emphasized the importance of measuring changes in the frequency of a response over time. In most cases, the measurement of response rate has been the analytical unit in operant research. Despite this emphasis, behavioural and pharmacological analyses have been conducted with other measures of behaviour such as the time between successive responses (interresponse time), as well as with other properties of the response such as force, location and duration. Due primarily to the historical emphasis on response rate, as well as to the fact that other properties of responses can also be controlled by schedules of reinforcement, the majority of research summarized in this chapter is based on experiments that analysed schedule-controlled response rate.

Under most conditions, behaviourally relevant consequences occur intermittently. Although it may appear paradoxical, behaviour is actually strengthened and intensified by carefully scheduled intermittent, rather than continuous, reinforcement. Properties of behaviour which have useful analytical dimensions, such as rate and patterning in time, can only be seen under conditions where consequent events are intermittently scheduled. Most schedules are variations on conditions that arrange for a consequent event to follow a response after a specified number of previous responses (*ratio* schedules) or after the passage of a certain period of time (*interval* schedules). Under both ratio and interval schedules, reinforcement can be arranged to follow a fixed or variable number of responses or a fixed or variable period of time. Under a *fixed-ratio* schedule, for example, reinforcement occurs following every *n*th response; under a *variable-ratio* schedule the number of responses required to obtain reinforcement varies around some average. *Fixed-interval* schedules reinforce the first response after a specified period of time has elapsed; with the *variable-interval* schedule, this time period varies. Figure 2.1 shows characteristic patterns of responding obtained under these schedules. Under the fixed-ratio schedule, responding follows an initial pause after each reinforcement and then occurs at a very high and sustained rate until the fixed-ratio requirement is completed and reinforcement occurs. High response rates are also maintained under the variable-ratio schedule but, depending on the parameter value of the ratio, pauses do not occur following reinforcement. Under the fixed-interval schedule there is a gradual transition from a period of no responding following reinforcement to a period with an intermediate rate of responding that is then followed by a higher response rate that persists until food is delivered. The variable-interval schedule produces a steady rate of responding with few pauses following reinforcement.

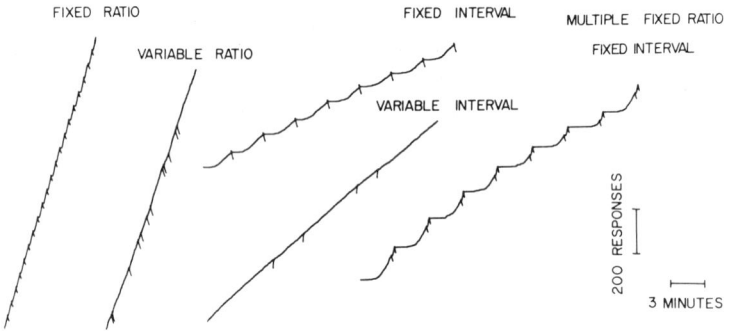

Fig. 2.1 Cumulative records depicting characteristic performances maintained under various schedules of reinforcement. Abscissa: time; ordinate: cumulative responses. Diagonal marks on the record indicate reinforcement.

Source: Barrett (1978).

In addition to basic interval and ratio schedules, other conditions can be arranged where reinforcement follows a response which occurs after a specified period of time has elapsed since the last response (differential reinforcement of low-rate schedule) or when the interval between successive responses is less than a certain time (differential reinforcement of high-rate schedule). Schedules can also be arranged in many different ways to operate sequentially or simultaneously and can be correlated with distinctive stimuli. For example, under the *multiple* schedule shown in Figure 2.1, a fixed-interval schedule was correlated with a red stimulus and a fixed-ratio schedule with a blue stimulus. Responding by the subject (a pigeon in this case) during each stimulus was appropriate to the schedule in effect and resembled that seen when each schedule was studied in isolation. Multiple schedules permit the study of different rates and patterns in a single subject within a relatively short period of time. Later in this chapter we will see that such schedules can provide useful information for understanding the effects of drugs on behaviour.

Schedules of reinforcement allow us to establish reliable quantitative, reproducible features of behaviour and to examine behavioural processes which are of general importance. Thus, schedules are useful methodological tools for the analysis of behaviour and the study of other variables, such as drugs, that affect behaviour. Experimentation with schedules of reinforcement has been criticized frequently on the grounds that they are artificial and without a direct counterpart under non-laboratory conditions. Few reinforcers, it is sometimes stated, occur with the regularity of those studied under fixed-interval or fixed-ratio schedules. Although mostly true, arguments of this type miss the point. Experimentally arranged schedules illuminate and reveal important aspects about how behaviour has been and is controlled by its environment. Most laboratory conditions are 'artificial' to some extent, yet still provide valuable information that can be generalized to non-laboratory situations. Experimental progress in any field is based on the ability to establish reliably that which is of interest. Schedules of reinforcement have done this for the study of behaviour and have greatly added to our understanding of behavioural principles of drug action (Barrett, 1980; Sanger, 1981).

Schedules of reinforcement not only produce reproducible patterns of responding within a single subject, but can also generate comparable performances across species and types of reinforcers. Figure 2.2 shows comparable performances by a squirrel monkey, a rabbit and a pigeon maintained under a multiple fixed-ratio, fixed-interval schedule of food presentation. If one is interested in determining the behavioural effects of certain interventions in different species, whether behavioural or pharmacological, those interventions should initially be made under conditions that are as comparable as possible. The use of schedules to develop similar performances across different species provides an initial step in the study of comparative behavioural pharmacology.

Schedules also allow the experimenter to establish comparable

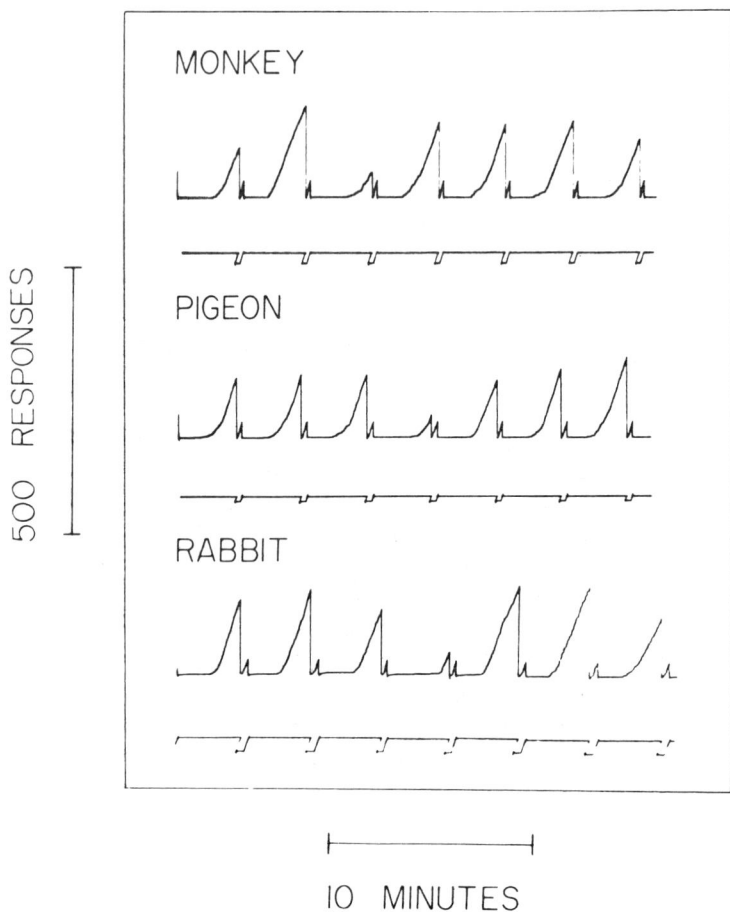

Fig. 2.2 Similar performances of a squirrel monkey, pigeon and rabbit under a multiple fixed-interval three-minute fixed-ratio thirty-response schedule of food presentation. The pen beneath each record was displaced during the fixed-ratio component; the response pen was reset after each food presentation. The pigeon pecked a Plexiglas key, whereas the monkey pressed and the rabbit lifted a lever. Note that patterns of responding were similar across the different species.

Source: Barrett and Tessel (1983).

behavioural performances maintained by different events. As we shall see, one question that has captured the attention of researchers in behavioural pharmacology has been whether the nature of the event that maintains behaviour (i.e. the organism's motivational state) can affect drug action. As with the study of drug effects in different species, it was important to conduct these experiments under conditions where the schedules were similar and the performances comparable. Under many conditions, the similar scheduling of different events can produce similar performances. Events as dissimilar as food or shock presentation, cocaine administration, or the termination of a stimulus in the presence of which shocks can occur maintain equivalent performances when studied under fixed-interval schedules. Schedules of reinforcement have not only proved useful for studying behavioural processes, but have also provided useful techniques for equating performances across species and types of maintaining events. Such features permit greater isolation and specificity in the identification of variables that potentially affect drug action.

Research in behavioural pharmacology has also relied heavily on schedules employing noxious stimuli such as electric shock. In most cases, electric shock has been used primarily to reduce or suppress responding by its presentation or to maintain responding by its postponement or removal. Electric shock is easily delivered, readily manipulated and quantitatively specifiable. However, other stimuli have also been used to suppress responding such as pressurized air and histamine injections. Experiments employing procedures in which behaviour is controlled by noxious stimuli have also contributed substantial information to an understanding of the mechanisms of the behavioural effects of drug.

The maintenance of behaviour by procedures where responding postpones or temporarily prevents the delivery of some event such as shock has typically been designated as avoidance. Under one type of avoidance procedure (Sidman, 1953), a response postpones a brief shock which is scheduled to recur regularly every t seconds. For example, in the absence of responding, shocks may be scheduled to occur every five seconds (the shock-shock interval); a response would postpone the next scheduled shock for twenty-five seconds (the response-shock interval). Traditionally, this non-discriminated or *continuous avoidance* procedure generates steady rates of responding and few shocks usually occur. With a different type of procedure, designated *discriminated avoidance* (Hoffman, 1966), a stimulus such as a tone or light usually precedes shock delivery and a response during the pre-shock stimulus terminates that stimulus and prevents shock; in the absence of a response, the stimulus usually terminates with shock delivery.

We have previously defined punishment as that process in which a reduction in responding is due to the response-dependent presentation of some event. Punishment is typically studied by establishing responding with a suitable reinforcer and then following all or some of the responses by shock or some other effective punishing event. Under most conditions, both the reinforcer and punisher are intermittently scheduled. Figure 2.3 shows data from a characteristic procedure for studying punishment which has been used frequently in behavioural pharmacology. In the presence of one stimulus, food is delivered under a fixed-interval schedule; food is also scheduled identically in the presence of a different stimulus but, in addition, every thirtieth response during this interval produces a brief electric shock. The degree of suppression depends on several factors such as the shock intensity, duration and frequency, as well as on the schedule maintaining responding and the degree of food deprivation. Procedures employing multiple schedules consisting of punished and unpunished responding are advantageous because they permit the study of variables of interest in the same individual organism within a relatively brief time period. There are many variations of punishment schedules. One of these, developed by Geller and Seifter (1960) and designated a 'conflict model', has been used extensively in behavioural pharmacology. In the presence of one stimulus, responding by a food-deprived subject produces food intermittently; periodically the stimulus changes and, for a brief period, each response produces both food and shock. Despite the higher frequency of food during this condition, responding is typically suppressed. Performances under this type of punishment schedule are quite sensitive to drugs from certain pharmacological classes and have been used quite successfully, for example, in detecting pre-clinically compounds with anti-anxiety properties.

A slightly different procedure which is usually referred to as conditioned suppression was first described by Estes and Skinner (1941). These researchers examined the effects of presenting a tone that terminated with electric shock to a rat responding under a fixed-interval food delivery schedule. After a number of tone-shock pairings, the onset of the tone suppressed ongoing operant responding.

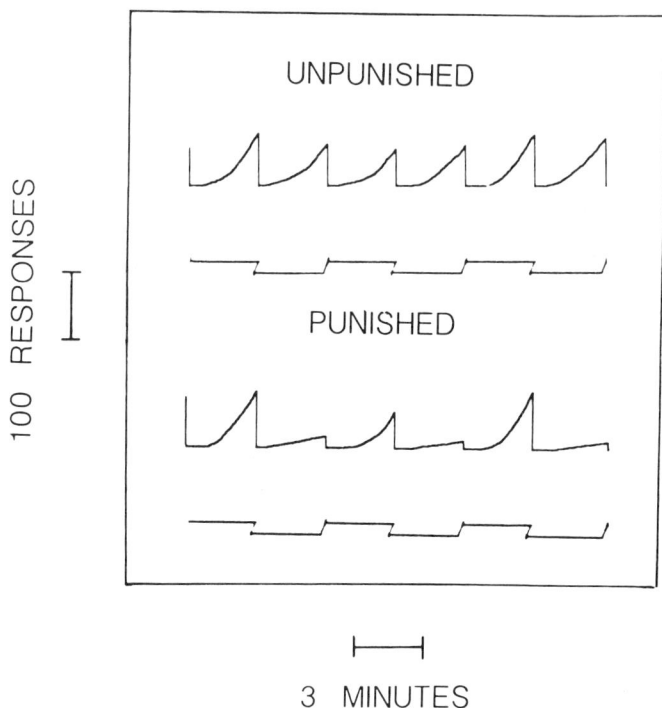

Fig. 2.3 Cumulative response records showing suppression of responding by punishment. Responding was maintained under a multiple three-minute fixed-interval schedule; the first response after three minutes produced food in the presence of each of two different visual stimuli (top record). When every thirtieth response during one component produced a 3 mA electric shock, responding during that component was suppressed (lower record).

Estes and Skinner designated the suppression as 'conditioned anxiety'. For rather obvious reasons, this procedure, with its attendant label 'anxiety', attracted a good deal of theoretical and experimental attention in early behavioural and psychopharmacological research (see Blackman, 1977 for a review of the behavioural literature). However, many of the initial studies using drugs produced inconsistent results. In addition, subsequent experiments showing suppression of ongoing food-maintained responding by stimuli paired with food posed difficulties of interpretation concerning the nature of suppression by both pre-food and pre-shock stimuli. Some of these issues have been addressed pharmacologically although, perhaps because of the combination of operant and respondent procedures, this procedure still does not enjoy widespread use.

Our discussion of the basic types of behaviour and overview of principles of the experimental analysis of behaviour are now complete. Although this treatment has been somewhat abbreviated, it should be clear that behaviour is controlled by multiple influences that act on existing behaviour as that behaviour is a product of the past. The principles and procedures reviewed thus far have provided a rich source of information and valuable techniques with which to ask questions about behavioural mechanisms of drug action. We are now in a position to review some of the effects of drugs on behaviour and to determine whether and how variables that influence behaviour also affect drug action.

Behavioural principles of drug action

Experiments with drugs and behaviour were initiated in Pavlov's laboratory during the time that work was first being conducted on the conditioned reflex (see Laties, 1979). However, the study of drugs on respondent behaviour has never developed to the degree seen with operant conditioning. Early experimentation with the effects of drugs on operant behaviour was initiated shortly after Skinner began his pioneering work (Skinner and Heron, 1937). More intensive studies using drugs and operant conditioning techniques were not conducted, however, until the use of chlorpromazine for managing psychotic behaviour in the 1950s prompted a direct interest in the use of behavioural techniques to assess and understand drug action. The remainder of this chapter will focus firstly on a brief description of the effects of drugs on respondent behaviour. It will then describe in greater detail research findings concerning the effects of drugs on operant behaviour from which most of our current understanding of behavioural principles of drug action have developed.

Drug effects on respondent behaviour

For the most part, experimentation with the effects of drugs on respondent behaviour has concentrated on the way in which drugs affect the acquisition process (i.e. learning) rather than on the alteration of established conditioned responses. This contrasts with most studies in behavioural pharmacology using operant procedures where the effects of drugs are examined on 'steady-state' behaviour. In one experiment that will serve to illustrate drug effects on a classically conditioned response, the effects of atropine were examined on the acquisition, maintenance and extinction of a classically conditioned discrimination in rabbits (Downs *et al.*, 1972). The nictitating membrane response (NMR) was conditioned to two tones that served as conditional stimuli. The unconditional stimulus consisted of a brief electric shock delivered to the skin of the paraorbital region. Shock delivery to this area elicits an unconditional response comprised of eyeball retraction which results in the passive extension of the nictitating membrane. During acquisition training one of the tones, each of which lasted 0.75 seconds, was immediately followed by shock, whereas the other tone terminated without shock delivery. Different groups of rabbits were trained with saline or subcutaneous injections of 10, 18 or 26 mg/kg of atropine. Compared with control groups treated with saline, all doses of atropine disrupted both acquisition and maintenance of the conditioned NMR response. Further, rabbits injected with 34 mg/kg of atropine prior to extinction showed fewer conditional eyeblink responses during extinction than saline-treated animals. Methylatropine, a quaternary ammonium derivative of atropine which exerts the same peripheral action as atropine but which does not pass readily through the blood-brain barrier, showed no retardant or decremental effects during either acquisition, maintenance or extinction, thereby indicating that the effects of atropine were centrally determined.

A series of experiments studying the effects of a wide variety of drugs has recently shown that the rate of acquisition of the NMR can be significantly increased by the hallucinogenic compound *d*-lysergic acid diethylamide (LSD). In one experiment, for example (Gimpl *et al.*, 1978), the NMR was conditioned to either a tone or light stimulus. Doses of LSD of 1−100 nmol/kg produced dose-dependent increases in the percentage of conditioned responses that occurred to both tone and light conditional stimuli. Figure 2.4 shows the effects of LSD on the conditioned NMR over the ten days of acquisition.

Both the rate of acquisition and asymptotic levels were affected. The bottom of this figure also indicates that LSD had no effect on responses to either tone or light stimuli when these were not paired with shock. Additional experiments which examined the frequency of responding to the conditional and unconditional stimuli alone (i.e. without pairing) demonstrated that LSD did not increase the frequency

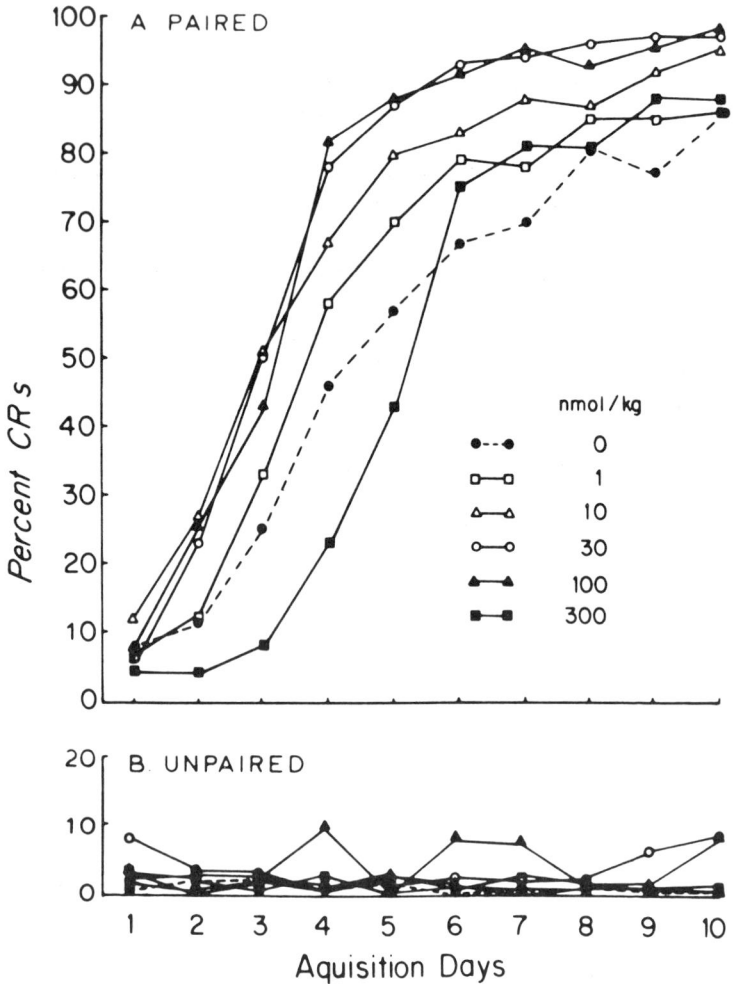

Fig. 2.4 Effects of LSD on acquisition of conditioned responses over days. Data are expressed as mean percentage of conditioned responses (CRs) on each of ten acquisition days. A: data for paired CS-UCS condition. B: data for an unpaired CS-UCS condition.

Source: Gimpl *et al.* (1978).

of the NMR, thereby indicating that the effects of LSD on acquisition were not attributable to conditioning artefacts (e.g. pseudoconditioning or sensitization). In a separate study, it was shown that LSD increased the frequency of a conditioned response to an extended range of stimulus intensities and also lowered the threshold for obtaining a conditioned response. Thus, it appeared that LSD was influencing acquisition by an effect on sensory processing (Gormezano *et al.*, 1980).

These studies are significant not only in demonstrating a facilatory effect on the acquisition of conditioned behaviour which may have implications for learning, but also because the experimenters utilized appropriate control groups to delineate the specificity of the drug effects. For example, another hallucinogen *dl*-2,5-dimethoxy-4-methylamphetamine (DOM) increased the rate of responding to the conditioned stimuli alone, thereby indicating an effect of this compound on 'non-associative factors' that are not necessarily involved in the acquisition process. Further studies using respondent conditioning procedures will probably yield additional information that is not only relevant and beneficial to an understanding of drug effects on respondent behaviour, but also useful for the development of general behavioural principles of drug action.

Operant behavioural pharmacology

This portion of the chapter will first describe some basic findings to illustrate some effects that drugs can have on operant behaviour. These results are then used as a focus for developing and elaborating the factors that may account for these effects.

Figure 2.5 shows some of the effects of ethanol and *d*-amphetamine on reinforced and punished behaviour of pigeons. In the top portion of this figure responding was maintained by food under a multiple fixed-interval, fixed-ratio schedule. Control or non-drug performances were similar to those shown earlier (Figure 2.1). After a 1.5 g/kg dose of ethanol, responding during the fixed-interval schedule was eliminated, whereas responding under the fixed ratio was increased. A similar finding with pentobarbital represented one of the first contributions to the behavioural pharmacology literature (Dews, 1955). The effects of *d*-amphetamine were just the opposite of those produced by ethanol: responding under the fixed-interval schedule was increased while performances under the fixed-ratio schedule were eliminated. Thus, the effects of both ethanol and amphetamine, although opposite in direction, depended on the schedule under which behaviour was maintained. Either drug could be categorized as 'stimulant' or 'depressant', depending on which behaviour was being studied.

In addition to demonstrating the importance of the schedule under

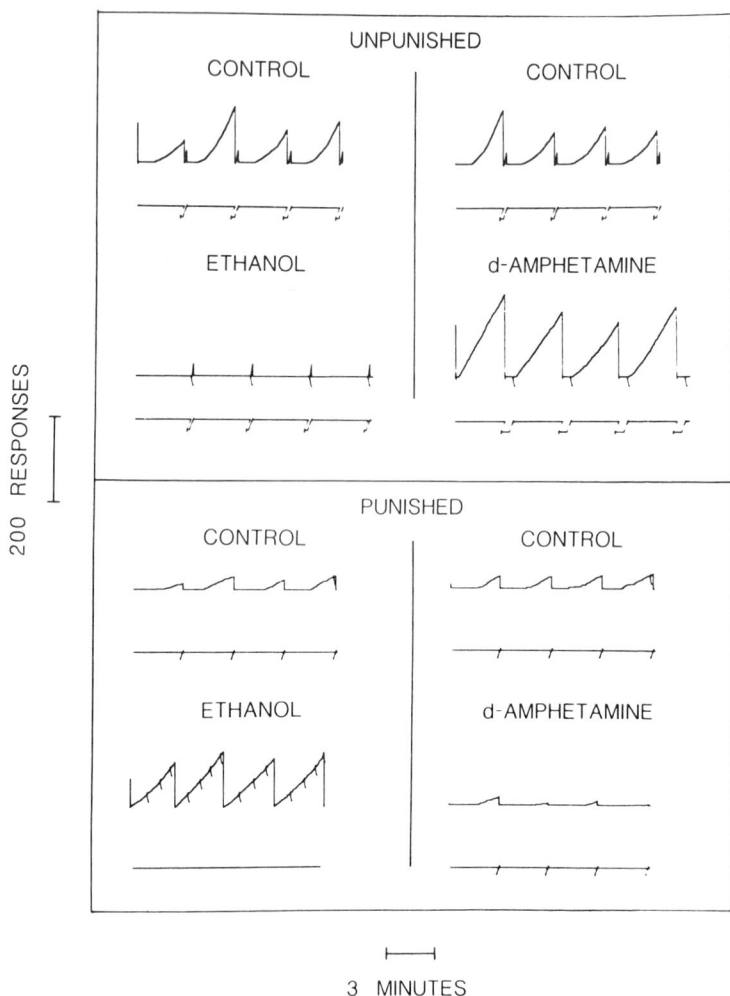

Fig. 2.5 Cumulative records illustrating effects of ethanol and amphetamine on unpunished and punished responding in pigeons. In the top portion the effects of ethanol (1.5 g/kg) and *d*-amphetamine (1.0 mg/kg) are shown on responding under a multiple fixed-interval fixed-ratio schedule of food presentation.

which behaviour occurs as a factor in drug action, this rather simple illustration has several other implications for evaluating and understanding the behavioural effects of drugs. For example, it is possible to eliminate explanations of effects of ethanol as due to motor incoordination. Although responding did not occur during the fixed-interval component, it is clear that the absence of responding was not because of motor impairment; response rates during the alternate fixed-ratio schedule component were actually *higher* than under control conditions. The high rates of responding under the fixed-ratio schedule (approximately three responses per second) actually require greater sustained response integration than the typically lower rates under the fixed interval. Similarly, explanations based on motivational decrements produced by a drug must acknowledge the selective, schedule-dependent nature of these changes. This is particularly relevant with amphetamine which, at high doses, can exert anorectic effects. Although fixed-ratio responding was decreased by amphetamine, responding still occurred at higher than control rates during the fixed-interval component. Thus, the behavioural effects of amphetamine and ethanol cannot easily be attributed to overall performance or motivational decrements, or to motor incapacitation. Although such factors may play a role at higher doses of these drugs, pronounced changes in behaviour occur at doses well below those that exert these effects. These results provide initial striking evidence, then, for the potentially important role of environmental factors in drug action.

There are numerous other instances in which the effects of drugs on behaviour are modified by non-pharmacological factors. An additional illustration is shown in the lower portion of Figure 2.5. In this case the effects of ethanol and *d*-amphetamine were studied on food-maintained behaviour reinforced under a fixed-interval schedule and punished by electric shock. Under these conditions ethanol increased responding, whereas amphetamine only decreased responding further. Thus, when behaviour maintained under a fixed interval is punished, the effects of ethanol and amphetamine are opposite to those found when behaviour is reinforced.

These results, together with those described earlier, demonstrate a significant contribution of behavioural variables to drug action. Although primarily illustrative, these studies not only highlight basic findings in behavioural pharmacology, but point to many of the complexities that must be dealt with when trying to account for and understand the effects of drugs on behaviour. There are obviously a host of variables that might potentially account for these effects; thus far, we have addressed only a few. In the remaining portions of this chapter we will explore those factors which have been suggested to be significant determinants of the behavioural effects of drugs.

Schedule-controlled response rate   The importance of the rate of responding that occurs in the absence of a drug was the first general principle to emerge in behavioural pharmacological research. Based on initial work by Dews (1958), this principle stems from the finding that the effects of certain doses of methamphetamine were related to the control rate at which behaviour occurred. Lower rates of responding under a fixed-interval fifteen-minute schedule were increased considerably, whereas higher rates occurring under a fixed-ratio schedule were decreased. These results are similar to those shown in the cumulative records in Figure 2.5 for amphetamine. This inverse relationship between response rate and the effects of amphetamines has been confirmed many times, in different species, and under a broad range of conditions (Dews and Wenger, 1977). Figure 2.6 shows a typical rate-dependent drug effect together with the usual method for analysing such effects. In this case, responding was maintained under a ten-minute fixed-interval schedule of food presentation. The interval was divided into four 150-second segments and response rates were calculated within each of these periods. Under control conditions, early in the interval (i.e. during the first 150 seconds), responding occurred at a low rate. As time elapsed, rates increased within successive intervals until a reasonably steady rate was reached that continued until food was delivered. When 3 mg/kg *d*-amphetamine was administered, the lower rates of responding (approximately 0.1 responses per second) in the early portion of the interval were increased to about 1000 per cent of control; higher rates (over one per second) of responding, however, were decreased to nearly 30% of control levels. Thus, the effects of amphetamine were related to the control rates of responding. This finding also appears to account for the effects shown earlier in this section (Figure 2.5) in which amphetamine increased the relatively lower rates of responding under the fixed-ratio schedule.

The significance of Dews' finding and the implications of rate-dependency for understanding drug effects on behaviour have been remarkable. For several years this principle served as a unifying theme

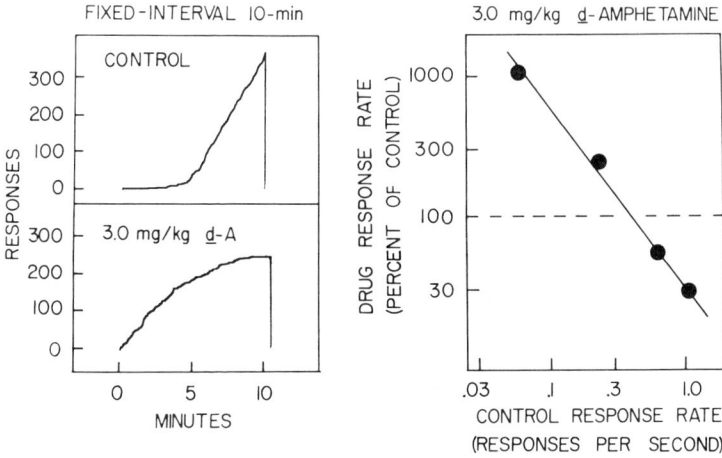

Fig. 2.6 Dependence of the effects of *d*-amphetamine sulphate on response rate. The figures on the left are cumulative records of responding under a ten-minute fixed-interval (FI) food schedule under control conditions (top) and after administration of 3 mg/kg *d*-amphetamine (bottom). Changes in response rates with *d*-amphetamine, expressed as a percentage of control, are shown in the log-log function on the right.

Source: Barrett (1980).

and organizing framework within which to approach, evaluate and understand the behavioural effects of drugs. The status of rate-dependency has been summarized several times (Dews and Wenger, 1977; Sanger and Blackman, 1976; Robbins, 1982) and, although some of the basic tenets have been questioned, the analysis and clarification of this principle continue to attract considerable interest.

Rate-dependent drug effects were once considered so pervasive that experiments which suggested factors other than rate-dependency were classified as 'exceptions' to the general principle. We have already seen two such exceptions in Figure 2.5 where the low rates of responding punished by electric shock were not increased by *d*-amphetamine and where ethanol increased the higher rates under the fixed-ratio schedule. Thus, several questions remain. Are only the effects of psychomotor stimulants on non-punished behaviour rate-dependent? Are the effects of sedative-hypnotic drugs such as the barbiturates independent of response rate or directly proportional to rate under conditions where behaviour is not punished? Does rate-dependency hold for some drugs under conditions where behaviour is reinforced and for other drugs when behaviour is punished? Unfortunately the answers to these and many other questions are not known at the present time.

There are, however, other schedule-related variables relevant to understanding the behavioural effects of drugs that have been studied. Many of these experiments were designed to analyse more fully the relative contribution of response rate or other variables to the behavioural effects of amphetamine. For example, under the multiple fixed-interval, fixed-ratio schedule the higher rates of responding under the fixed-ratio schedule result in a higher frequency of reinforcement. Under the fixed-interval schedule, however, reinforcement frequency is largely independent of response rate. Thus, perhaps some of the rate-dependent effect of amphetamine is related to the frequency of reinforcement. However, when experiments have examined different response rates maintained by equivalent frequencies of reinforcement, the effects appear more strongly related to response rate than reinforcement frequency. For example, MacPhail and Gollub (1975) used a three-component multiple schedule which, by reinforcing selected interresponse times, maintained three different rates of responding with similar frequencies of reinforcement. In this study, the effects of amphetamine depended more on control rate of responding than on the frequency of reinforcement.

Other experiments have not been as supportive of rate-dependency as an embracing principle in determining the behavioural effects of drugs (see below). However, an understanding and appreciation of the importance of response rate is essential not only for evaluating drug effects but for a proper assessment of the development of research in behavioural pharmacology. This principle has guided a vast amount of research and has, both directly and indirectly, allowed new principles to emerge which have shaped the current state of the field. One of the early 'exceptions' to rate-dependency was that drug effects are modified by the discriminative stimuli present when behaviour is occurring.

Discriminative stimuli Environmental stimuli present when a response is reinforced can acquire substantial control over behaviour. In most cases this control will be exerted by visual or auditory stimuli, although it is possible for a drug to acquire discriminative control over behaviour (see Chapter 3). This chapter has described several experiments using multiple schedules where visual stimuli have controlled different rates and patterns of responding. The rate and pattern of responding in the presence of discriminative stimuli depend on both the preceding history of reinforcement and on the current schedule conditions. One means by which drugs may affect behaviour is by modifying in some way the control exerted by discriminative stimuli. Experimental approaches to this issue are problematical, however, because the measurement of stimulus control depends on differential response rates in the presence of the different stimuli. As we have already seen, drug effects can be related to the control rate of responding and, under conditions where different rates are occurring, it is difficult to separate drug effects on response rate from those that may be ascribed to effects on stimulus control. For example, under a multiple schedule in which relatively high and low rates of responding occur in two components, amphetamine may decrease the higher rates and increase those that occur with a lower frequency. Can these effects be attributable to influences on rate of responding or, alternatively, to some disruption in the degree to which the discriminative stimuli control behaviour?

Several studies have demonstrated that the addition of discriminative stimuli or modifications in the physical properties of those stimuli (e.g. changes in stimulus intensity) can produce quantitative differences in the effects of a variety of drugs. In most instances, however, these manipulations have also altered the control rates of responding. Questions about the effects of drugs on stimulus control demand a separate analytical approach from those which have been used customarily to suggest the modification of drug action by discriminative stimuli. Some method for separating the effects of drugs on stimulus control from those on rate must be employed to resolve these issues satisfactorily. Techniques such as those based on sensory psychophysics and signal detection theory appear to be appropriate to answering questions of this type (Seiden and Dykstra, 1977).

A recent series of experiments using schedule-controlled procedures similar to those discussed in this chapter has examined the extent to which changes in rates of responding produced by drugs are due to changes in discriminative control (Katz, 1982, 1983). Response-rate changes and changes in stimulus control were assessed independently by a method similar to that used in signal detection analysis. In these experiments pigeons were trained to respond to one of two coloured keys depending on whether a light which provided general illumination (houselight) was present or absent. When the houselight was illuminated, pecks on a red key produced food under a five-minute fixed-interval schedule (S^D responses); pecks on an amber key in the presence of the houselight did not produce food (S^Δ responses). When the houselight was off, pecks on the amber key produced food under the fixed-interval schedule, and pecks on the red key did not. Thus, whether responding on the red or amber key was reinforced was conditional upon the presence or absence of the houselight. The degree to which the houselight controlled the distribution of responses on either the red or amber keys could vary independently of the rate with which responding on those keys occurred.

Stimulus control was measured by a method analogous to that used for measuring sensitivity in signal detection analysis. The measure of sensitivity or stimulus control (A') relates the tendency to respond appropriately when the houselight is present with the tendency to respond inappropriately in the absence of the houselight (i.e. to respond as though the houselight were present). A high degree of control is indicated by a high rate of responding on the red key in the presence of the houselight and a low rate of responding on the red key in the absence of the houselight.

Performances under non-drug conditions indicated near perfect control by the houselight. Responding on the S^D key occurred at a high rate, whereas responding on the S^Δ key was minimal. Intermediate doses of all these drugs typically increased the higher response rates on the S^D key and produced relatively little effect on the S^Δ key responses. The highest dose of each of the drugs markedly decreased all responding. Despite these rather large changes in responding, most doses of the drugs had little effect on stimulus control. Only the highest doses, which also decreased responding, disrupted stimulus control; even then, these were relatively small decreases. This study demonstrates that drug effects on schedule-controlled behaviour occur at doses that do not modify the control of behaviour by visual discriminative stimuli.

Clearly, much additional work needs to be conducted before more general statements can be made about stimulus control and drug effects. The process of discrimination, like the processes of reinforcement and punishment, is exceedingly complex and demands a rigorous, consistent methodology. Refinements and application of newer techniques promise to extend our understanding of the role that discriminative stimuli play in influencing the behavioural effects of drugs.

Nature of the event maintaining behaviour   As we have seen in early portions of this chapter, it is possible to maintain behaviour by a wide variety of consequent events. Questions pertaining to the contribution of the type of event as a potential influence on drug action have been raised since behavioural pharmacology was first established as a formal discipline. Part of the importance of such factors is attributable to the fact that theories of motivational determinants of behaviour were dominant during the early phases of behavioural research using drugs and such factors were often incorporated into accounts of drug action. According to such views, compounds which alleviated anxiety or minimized the influence of noxious environmental conditions should affect behaviour controlled by food differently from that controlled by shock. Some studies did demonstrate that certain drugs produced effects on food-maintained behaviour that differed from those found on behaviour controlled, for example, by shock avoidance. However, many of these studies neglected to control for the influence of response rate so that any differential drug effects may have been due to the different rates of responding rather than to the types of maintaining events. When more comparable performances controlled by different events were established, it appeared that the schedule-controlled rate and pattern of responding were more important than the maintaining event. For example, chlorpromazine had similar rate-decreasing effects on responding controlled by food or by termination of a stimulus-shock complex (Kelleher and Morse, 1964). The finding that the antipsychotic compounds decrease responding and that other drugs such as amphetamine increase responding controlled by different events has been confirmed in several experiments (McKearney and Barrett, 1978). Subsequent studies with a wider variety of drugs and a range of performances controlled by food or shock presentation, stimulus-shock termination or drug administration, however, have shown that under many conditions the type of maintaining event can be an important factor in determining the effects of drugs on behaviour (see reviews by Barrett, 1981; Barrett and Katz, 1981). A review of one of these studies in detail illustrates this point.

  Performances of squirrel monkeys were maintained by food or shock presentation under a multiple five-minute fixed-interval schedule (Barrett, 1976). Lever pressing maintained by response-produced shock was established by procedures discussed earlier in this chapter; i.e. most monkeys were trained initially under a shock-postponement schedule. Shock intensity was adjusted to establish comparable rates and patterns of responding maintained by food and shock. Under these conditions chlordiazepoxide, pentobarbital and ethanol increased responding maintained by food but only decreased responding maintained by shock (Figure 2.7). Cocaine, however, increased responding maintained by both events. In a more extensive examination of the effects of chlordiazepoxide on food and shock-maintained responding, control rates were manipulated so that rates of responding maintained by food were both higher and lower than those maintained by shock. Despite these differences in rates, the effects of chlordiazepoxide were qualitatively similar to those found when rates were equal. Thus, under these conditions, the effects of chlordiazepoxide were more related to the type of maintaining event than to the rate at which responding occurred.

There is now little doubt that the effects of many drugs can be determined by the type of event that maintains behaviour. For the most part, studies have compared the effects of drugs on performances maintained by appetitive events with those maintained by noxious consequences. Far fewer experiments have examined drug effects on performances controlled by events such as food presentation, brain stimulation, drug administration, or by the postponement of shock or drug injections. Studies comparing similar performances maintained by food delivery or drug administration would be important in determining whether drugs exert uniform effects on behaviour maintained by traditional appetitive consequences. At the present time it is clear that the types of consequences maintaining behaviour can qualitatively affect the way behaviour is changed by certain drugs. It is not clear what factors are responsible for different drug effects. Ultimately, however, it should be possible to delineate more precisely those factors that contribute to drug effects that depend on the type of maintaining event.

Behavioural and pharmacological history   The contribution of prior experience to current behaviour has been discussed earlier in this chapter. In this section we will see that prior behavioural history, i.e. the consequences of past behaviour, can also play a substantial role in determining the effects of a number of drugs on behaviour. In addition, we will discuss experiments that indicate that prior experience with one drug can also directly influence the manner in which behaviour is changed by other drugs. These findings have important

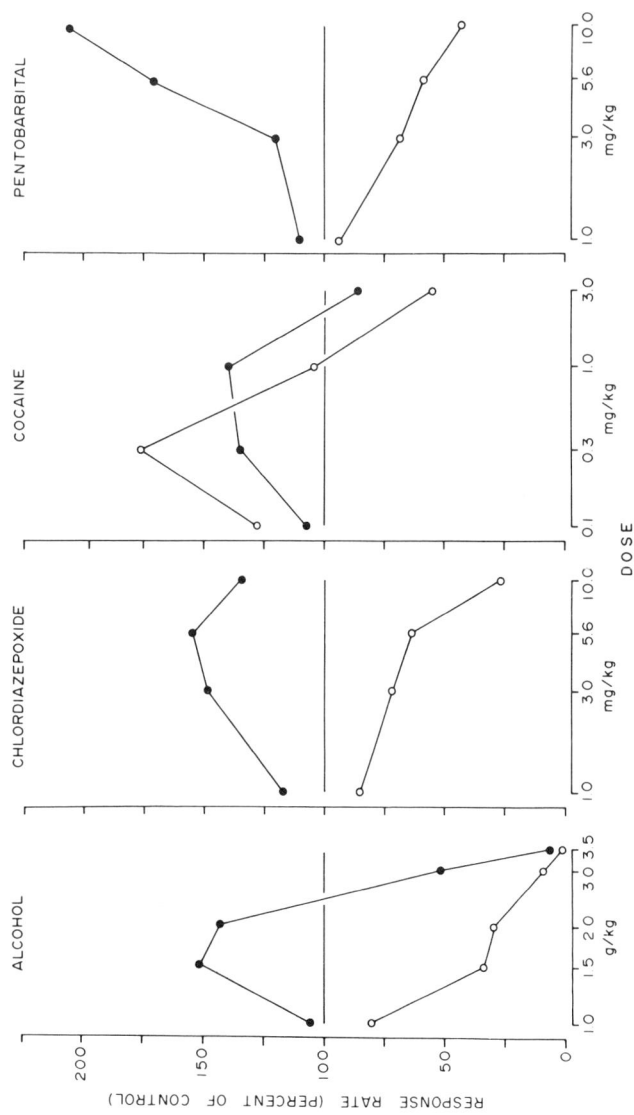

Fig. 2.7 Effects of alcohol, chlordiazepoxide, cocaine and pentobarbital on overall rates of responding under a multiple five-minute fixed-interval schedule of food or shock presentation. Each point represents the mean of at least two determinations for each of three subjects expressed as the percentage of control response rate. Filled circles represent responding maintained by food, open circles responding maintained by shock.

Source: Barrett (1976).

implications for establishing basic behavioural principles of drug action and have direct relevance for understanding potential factors involved in drug abuse.

An early experiment by Terrace (1963) demonstrated that the conditions under which a visual discrimination is established can substantially alter the effects of the antipsychotic drug chlorpromazine and the antidepressant compound imipramine. Key pecking by pigeons was maintained by providing food under a schedule when the stimulus on the key consisted of a vertical line (S^D); key pecking was not reinforced in the presence of a horizontal line (S^Δ). One group of pigeons was trained directly on the line discrimination where many responses occurred to both S^D and S^Δ, though, eventually, S^Δ responses declined to near zero. A second group of pigeons was trained first on a red-green discrimination 'without errors'. This procedure, developed by Terrace, permitted a perfect discrimination to be established (i.e. responding in the presence of S^D, but no responding to S^Δ) by first training pigeons to peck in the presence of the red keylight. Once responding was firmly established, the green stimulus was presented briefly and its duration was gradually lengthened to equal that of the red stimulus. This technique establishes red-green discrimination without any responses occurring to S^Δ (an 'errorless discrimination' procedure). With the errorless-trained group, the vertical and horizontal lines were then superimposed on the red-green stimuli respectively, and the colours were gradually faded out; no responses ever occurred with this group when the horizontal line (S^Δ) was present. Thus, at the time drugs were administered one group had a prior history of responding to S^Δ, whereas the other group did not; little or no responding occurred to S^Δ in either group. Both chlorpromazine and imipramine increased responding to S^Δ only in those pigeons trained in the conventional manner (i.e. with 'errors'). Increases in responding during S^Δ did not occur at any dose with those pigeons trained 'without errors'. In this experiment, then, the previous training conditions appeared to produce terminal behavioural performances that were differentially sensitive to the effects of drugs.

Other studies have also demonstrated the importance of prior behavioural experience in determining drug effects. In one experiment (Barrett, 1977) squirrel monkeys were initially trained under a fixed-interval schedule of food delivery. Subsequently, when every thirtieth response during each interval was followed by electric shock, responding was suppressed. As discussed previously, d-amphetamine

(0.01–0.56 mg/kg) did not increase this punished behaviour (left panel, Figure 2.8). These monkeys were then trained under a shock-postponement schedule for approximately two weeks and were then returned to the punishment schedule where, at the time amphetamine was again administered, performances were comparable to those during the first phase. In marked contrast to the effects obtained with amphetamine initially, this drug now produced sizeable increases in punished responding (right panel, Figure 2.8). Interpolated training under the avoidance schedule completely reversed the behavioural effects of amphetamine.

These experiments, plus others (McKearney and Barrett, 1978),

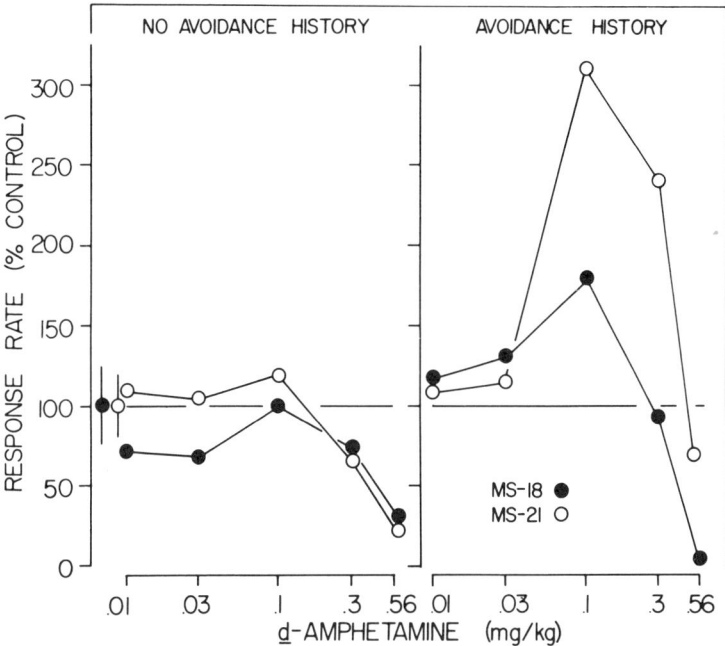

Fig. 2.8 Modification of the effects of *d*-amphetamine on punished responding by behavioural history in two monkeys (MS 18, MS 21). The left portion of the figure shows the effects of *d*-amphetamine on punished responding prior to training under a shock-postponement or avoidance schedule. In marked contrast to the effects obtained initially, *d*-amphetamine produced substantial increases in punished responding after the avoidance history.

Source: adapted from Barrett (1977).

provide substantial evidence that prior behavioural experience can override the contribution of current environmental conditions and reverse the more characteristic effects that a drug will have on behaviour. Clearly, the effects of some drugs appear quite malleable and sensitive to behavioural experience. Principles derived from such studies not only contribute to a description of behavioural principles influencing drug action but may also contribute to an understanding of aspects of drug abuse. For example, if the effects a drug has on behaviour are related to its abuse potential, then experiential factors which directly alter the behavioural effects of these drugs may play a direct role in drug-abuse liability.

Drug effects on behaviour can be altered not only by prior behavioural experience, but also by prior experience with other drugs. This effect is to be distinguished from situations where *tolerance* develops to the effects of a drug when that drug is administered repeatedly and higher doses are required to produce similar behavioural effects. Prior drug experience, as discussed here, also differs from *behavioural tolerance* in which behavioural and/or environmental factors influence the development of pharmacological tolerance (e.g. Corfield-Sumner and Stolerman, 1978).

One experiment showing that a history with one drug can alter the effects of a drug from a different pharmacological class was conducted with squirrel monkeys under a procedure in which responding maintained under a stimulus-shock termination schedule was punished by shock presentation (Glowa and Barrett, 1983). With one group of monkeys the effects of pentobarbital were examined first; with a second group, the effects of pentobarbital were determined after those of morphine. In both groups of monkeys, complete dose-effect curves were obtained with one drug before the other drug was studied. Pentobarbital increased responding when it was the first drug studied. When the effects of pentobarbital were determined after those of morphine, however, pentobarbital did not increase punished responding. Thus, prior experience with morphine, which did not increase responding, appeared to prevent the rate-increasing effects of pentobarbital.

Such experiments demonstrate an important role for prior drug experience in contributing to the effects a drug can have on behaviour. Studies with drug self-administration have also indicated that prior drug history can influence whether a drug will be self-administered. Findings of this nature, together with those discussed previously in this chapter, point rather convincingly to the widespread and fundamental importance of behavioural and environmental factors as determinants of drug action.

It is important to appreciate the fact that with both pharmacological and behavioural history, the influence of these previous experiences appears to persist long after the initial conditions were in effect. Current features of ongoing behaviour such as rate or patterning showed no indication of the effects of prior experience until a drug was administered. Thus, residual influences produced by previous experience appear to continue for some time and produce relatively enduring changes in drug action. At present, little is known about how long such changes continue, about conditions which may reinstate initial drug effects, or about the specific mechanisms through which prior behavioural and pharmacological history produce their effects. These are experimental questions, the answers to which will undoubtedly expand our understanding of behavioural and pharmacological determinants of drug action.

Environmental context   The preceding section on behavioural and pharmacological history has indicated that temporally remote factors which are no longer in effect can continue to influence drug effects on behaviour. In this section we will examine how conditions that are in effect simultaneously or sequentially also modify the behavioural effects of drugs.

Under multiple schedules of reinforcement, changes in the consequences of responding in one component can often affect behaviour in an alternate component, even though the latter conditions have not changed (e.g. behavioural contrast). Similar factors can also influence the way behaviour is changed by drugs. For example, *d*-amphetamine did not increase punished responding of squirrel monkeys when this behaviour occurred during one component of a multiple schedule that alternated with extinction (McKearney and Barrett, 1975). However, when the extinction component was replaced with a shock-postponement schedule, *d*-amphetamine produced sizeable increases in punished behaviour, even though punished performances did not change (Figure 2.9). Thus, conditions that affect behaviour in one context can produce changes in the way a drug affects behaviour under a different condition. This result is similar to that discussed in the previous section where the effects of *d*-amphetamine on punished behaviour were altered by prior experience. The finding that this

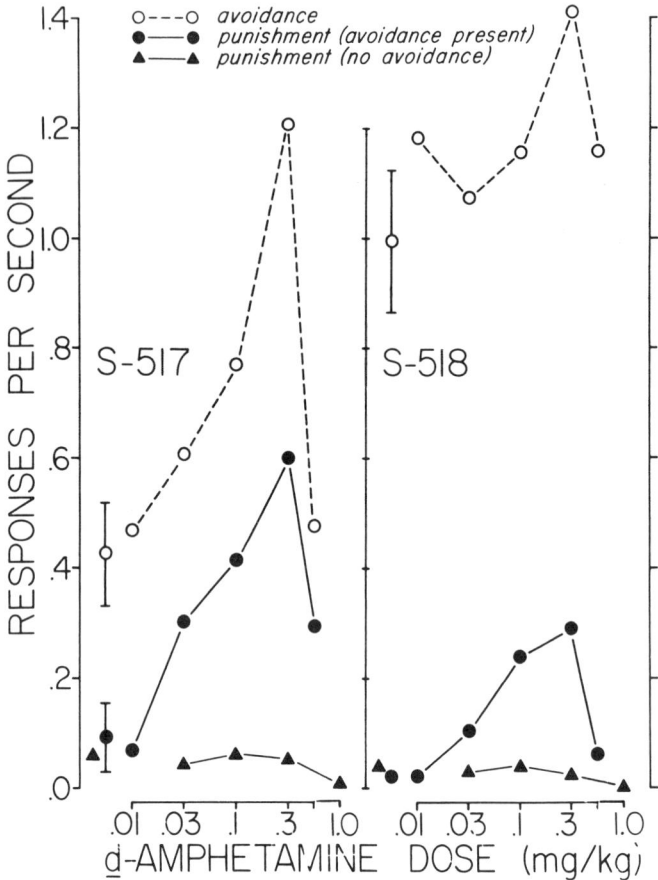

Fig. 2.9   Effects of *d*-amphetamine on punished responding of two squirrel monkeys under a multiple schedule when this behaviour alternated with an extinction component in which responding had no consequences (triangles) and when this component was replaced by an avoidance schedule (filled circles). *d*-Amphetamine increased punished responding only when the avoidance schedule was in effect.

Source: McKearney and Barrett (1975).

exposure can occur under a multiple schedule suggests that influences that change behaviour and drug action under a multiple schedule may persist beyond the immediate context in which those effects took place. Further, such factors may continue to influence drug effects even when they are no longer part of the current environment.

Summary and conclusions

This chapter has focused on basic principles of behaviour and on the contribution of those principles to the study and understanding of the behavioural effects of drugs. There has been a continuing and beneficial interplay between the experimental analysis of behaviour and behavioural pharmacology. Many of the fundamental principles of behaviour, such as reinforcement and punishment, and the variables of which behaviour is a function, such as prior history, are also fundamental determinants of the behavioural effects of drugs. Principles important for an understanding of behaviour are also important for an understanding of the behavioural effects of drugs. The experimental analysis of behaviour has clarified and elaborated certain basic principles which have general importance and permit precise, analytical approaches to revealing behavioural mechanisms of drug action.

The experiments described in this chapter demonstrate that a drug is not simply a molecule with static, unitary behavioural effects. The same dose of a drug can exert an array of effects on behaviour depending on the immediate consequences of responding, the prior experience of the organism and the total environmental context in which the behaviour takes place. Dramatic, qualitative modifications in the behavioural effects of drugs produced by such factors indicate that the mechanisms by which these effects are produced are quite powerful. The range of conditions under which such effects occur and the variety of drugs with which these effects can be demonstrated suggest that environmental determinants of the behavioural effects of drugs are not of limited generality. Although much additional work remains, it would appear that the framework for a sound discipline with both fundamental and practical significance has taken shape. Subsequent experimentation will undoubtedly establish new principles and clarify many of the questions posed in the present chapter.

References

Baez, L. A. (1976) Effects of drugs on arousal and consummatory behavior. In S. D. Glick and J. Goldfarb (eds) *Behavioral Pharmacology*. St Louis: C. V. Mosby, pp. 140–75.

Barrett, J. E. (1976) Effects of alcohol, chlordiazepoxide, cocaine and pentobarbital on responding maintained under fixed-interval schedules of food or shock presentation. *Journal of Pharmacology and Experimental Therapeutics 196*: 605–15.

Barrett, J. E. (1977) Behavioral history as a determinant of the effects of d-amphetamine on punished behavior. *Science 198*: 67–9.

Barrett, J. E. (1978) Learning theories: operant paradigm. In G. U. Balis, L. Wurmser, E. McDaniel and R. G. Grennell (eds) *The Psychiatric Foundations of Medicine*. Woburn, Mass.: Butterworth, pp. 73–108.

Barrett, J. E. (1980) Behavioral pharmacology: recent developments and new trends. *Trends in Pharmacological Sciences 1*: 215–18.

Barrett, J. E. (1981) Differential drug effects as a function of the controlling consequences. In T. Thompson and C. E. Johanson (eds) *Behavioral Pharmacology of Human Drug Dependence*, NIDA Research Monograph no. 37. Washington, DC: US Government Printing Office, pp. 159–81.

Barrett, J. E. and Katz, J. L. (1981) Drug effects on behaviors maintained by different events. In T. Thompson, P. B. Dews and W. A. McKim (eds) *Advances in Behavioral Pharmacology*. Vol. III. New York: Academic Press, pp. 119–68.

Barrett, J. E. and Tessel, R. E. (1983) Behavioral pharmacology of drugs affecting norepinephrine transmission. In M. G. Ziegler and C. R. Lake (eds) *Norepinephrine: Clinical Aspects*. Baltimore: Williams and Wilkins.

Blackman, D. E. (1974) *Operant Conditioning*. London: Methuen.

Blackman, D. E. (1977) Conditioned suppression and the effects of classical conditioning on operant behavior. In W. K. Honig and J. E. R. Staddon (eds) *Handbook of Operant Behavior*. Englewood Cliffs, NJ: Prentice-Hall, pp. 340–63.

Corfield-Sumner, P. K. and Stolerman, I. P. (1978) Behavioral tolerance. In D. E. Blackman and D. J. Sanger (eds) *Contemporary Research in Behavioral Pharmacology*. New York: Plenum Press, pp. 391–448.

Dews, P. B. (1955) Studies on behavior. I. Differential sensitivity to pentobarbital of pecking performance in pigeons depending on the schedule of reward. *Journal of Pharmacology and Experimental Therapeutics 113*: 393–401.

Dews, P. B. (1958) Studies on behavior. IV. Stimulant actions of methamphetamine. *Journal of Pharmacology and Experimental Therapeutics 122*: 137–47.

Dews, P. B. and Wenger, G. R. (1977) Rate-dependency of the behavioral effects of amphetamine. In T. Thompson and P. B. Dews (eds) *Advances in Behavioral Pharmacology*. Vol. 1. New York: Academic Press, pp. 167–227.

Downs, D., Cardozo, C., Schneiderman, N., Yehle, A. L., Van Dercar, D. H. and Zwilling, G. (1972) Central effects of atropine upon aversive classical conditioning in rabbits. *Psychopharmacologia 23*: 319–33.

Estes, W. K. and Skinner, B. F. (1941) Some quantitative properties of anxiety. *Journal of Experimental Psychology 29*: 390–400.

Ferster, C. B. and Skinner, B. F. (1957) *Schedules of Reinforcement*. New York: Appleton-Century-Crofts.

Geller, I. and Seifter, J. (1960) The effects of meprobamate, barbiturates, *d*-amphetamine and promazine on experimentally induced confier in the rat. *Psychopharmacologia I*: 482–91.

Gimpl, M. P., Gormezano, I. and Harvey, J. A. (1978) Effects of LSD on learning as measured by classical conditioning of the rabbit nictitating membrane response. *Journal of Pharmacology and Experimental Therapeutics 208*: 330–4.

Glowa, J. R. and Barrett, J. E. (1983) Drug history modifies the behavioral effects of pentobarbital. *Science 220*: 333–5.

Gormezano, I., Harvey, J. A. and Aycock, E. (1980) Sensory and associative effects of LSD on classical appetitive conditioning of the rabbit jaw movement response. *Psychopharmacology 70*: 137–43.

Hoffman, H. S. (1966) The analysis of discriminated avoidance. In W. K. Honig (ed.) *Operant Behavior: Areas of Research and Application*. New York: Appleton-Century-Crofts, pp. 499–530.

Katz, J. L. (1982) Drug effects and stimulus control of responding. I. Independent assessment of effects on response rates and stimulus control. *Journal of Pharmacology and Experimental Therapeutics 223*: 617–23.

Katz, J. L. (1983) Effects of drugs on stimulus control of behavior. II. Dependence of effect on degree of stimulus control. *Journal of Pharmacology and Experimental Therapeutics 226*: 756–63.

Kelleher, R. T. and Morse, W. H. (1964) Escape behavior and punished behavior. *Federation Proceedings 23*: 808–17.

Laties, V. G. (1979) I. V. Zavodskii and the beginnings of behavioral pharmacology: an historical note and translation. *Journal of the Experimental Analysis of Behavior 32*: 463–72.

McKearney, J. W. and Barrett, J. E. (1975) Punished behavior: increases in responding after *d*-amphetamine. *Psychopharmacologia 41*: 23–6.

McKearney, J. W. and Barrett, J. E. (1978) Schedule-controlled behavior and the effects of drugs. In D. E. Blackman and D. J. Sanger (eds) *Contemporary Research in Behavioral Pharmacology*. New York: Plenum Press, pp. 1–68.

MacPhail, R. C. and Gollub, L. R. (1975) Separating the effects of response rate and reinforcement frequency in the rate-dependent effects of amphetamine and scopolamine on the schedule-controlled performance of rats and pigeons. *Journal of Pharmacology and Experimental Therapeutics 194*: 332–42.

Miczek, K. A. and Barry, H., III (1976) Pharmacology of sex and aggression. In S. D. Glick and J. Goldfarb (eds) *Behavioral Pharmacology*. St Louis: C. V. Mosby, pp. 176–257.

Morse, W. H. (1966) Intermittent reinforcement. In W. K. Honig (ed.) *Operant Behavior: Areas of Research and Application*. New York: Appleton-Century-Crofts, pp. 52–108.

Pavlov, I. P. (1927) *Conditioned Reflexes*. London: Oxford University Press.

Robbins, T. W. (1977) A critique of the methods available for the measurement of spontaneous motor activity. In L. L. Iversen, S. D. Iversen and S. H. Snyder (eds) *Handbook of Psychopharmacology*. Vol. 7. New York: Plenum Press, pp. 37–82.

Robbins, T. W. (1982) Behavioral determinants of drug action: rate dependency revisited. In S. J. Cooper (ed.) *Theory in Psychopharmacology*. New York: Academic Press, pp. 1–63.

Sanger, D. J. (1981) The role of operant behaviour in the pharmacology laboratory. In C. M. Bradshaw, E. Szabadi and C. F. Lowe (eds) *Quantification of Steady State Operant Behaviour*. Amsterdam: Elsevier, pp. 233–47.

Sanger, D. J. and Blackman, D. E. (1976) Rate-dependent effects of drugs: a review of the literature. *Pharmacology, Biochemistry and Behavior 4*: 73–83.

Seiden, L. S. and Dykstra, L. A. (1977) *Psychopharmacology: A Biochemical and Behavioral Approach*. New York: Van Nostrand Reinhold.

Sidman, M. (1953) Avoidance conditioning with brief shock and no exteroceptive warning signal. *Science 118*: 157–8.

Skinner, B. F. (1938) *The Behavior of Organisms*. New York: Appleton-Century-Crofts.

Skinner, B. F. and Heron, W. T. (1937) Effects of caffeine and benzedrine upon conditioning and extinction. *Psychological Record 1*: 340–6.

Terrace, H. S. (1963) Errorless discrimination learning in the pigeon: effects of chlorpromazine and imipramine. *Science 140*: 318–19.

3 Internal stimulus effects of drugs

I. P. Stolerman

Introduction

It is important to recognize and investigate the internal stimulus properties of drugs if we are to fully understand their psychological and behavioural effects. Drugs may serve as internal stimuli in many different situations and not only when programmed to do so for experimental purposes.

The mainstream of behavioural pharmacology has involved studying the effects of drugs on a wide variety of conditioned and unconditioned behavioural responses. The preceding chapter by J. E. Barrett includes an account of drug effects on behaviours established by the techniques of operant conditioning; typically, the effects of drugs are demonstrated by first developing a stable baseline of responding according to the requirements of a schedule of reinforcement, and then observing how this behaviour changes when a drug is administered. In such circumstances, the drugs serve as independent variables which alter the characteristics, notably response rates, of the schedule-controlled behaviour. The schedules use external stimuli such as cue lights, audible tones, food or shock reinforcers to maintain the behavioural baseline prior to the administration of drugs.

Increasingly often, situations have been studied where drugs are not merely independent variables but form an integral part of the controlling schedule of reinforcement, to the extent that the schedule-controlled behaviour would never emerge in the absence of the drug. In such circumstances, the effects of drugs serve the same functions in relation to behaviour as conventional external stimuli (e.g. a drug is given when a cue light or food reinforcer would otherwise be presented). It is known that the conventional environmental stimuli can influence operant behaviour by exerting discriminative, reinforcing or aversive effects, and drugs can fill all these functions by acting as internal stimuli. In classical conditioning, previously 'neutral' stimuli come to act as conditioned stimuli and to influence behaviour through their association with various unconditioned stimuli; drugs too have the ability to serve as the conditioned or unconditioned stimuli in classical conditioning. The whole area, regardless of whether an operant or classical conditioning technique is used, forms the distinct part of behavioural pharmacology which is generally known as the study of the stimulus properties of drugs.

Research where drugs serve as internal stimuli can help to reduce the gap between experimental work and clinical psychopharmacology, and may shed light on how internal stimuli control normal behaviour. Patients often describe mental illness and the effects of drugs in terms of how they feel. The use of animal subjects generally makes it very difficult to interpret drug effects in terms of feelings, moods and motivational states. The study of ways in which drugs serve as identifiable internal stimuli, producing effects which the animal detects and then acts upon, provides some of the most promising approaches to bridging this gap between clinical and animal work. Thus, animals may be trained to behave one way when a particular drug is administered and in a different way in the absence of the drug; it then becomes possible to assess whether a different drug produces effects which the animal perceives as like those of the drug used for training. There are important applications for the use of drugs as stimuli in areas such as the development of new drugs, in studies of the neurochemical mode of action of drugs in the body, and in the understanding of clinical problems such as drug addiction.

This chapter is principally concerned with those stimulus properties of drugs which have been investigated in greatest depth, namely their discriminative and motivational effects. The aim is to acquaint readers with the basic characteristics of the situations in which these effects occur, their uses and limitations in psychopharmacology, and their applications to some clinical problems. The development of this

field of study has led to new questions being asked about the fundamental behavioural processes involved, and promises to advance our
knowledge of the relationships between subjective sensations, moods
and emotion on the one hand, and overt behaviour on the other.

Drugs as discriminative stimuli

Basic characteristics of the paradigm

A discriminative stimulus may be defined as an environmental event
which indicates the occasions on which a particular type of behaviour
is reinforced. For example, a rat may be able to obtain food reinforcers by pressing a bar when an audible tone is present, but
pressing the bar in the absence of the tone is not reinforced. If the rat
acquires the appropriate behaviour, the tone is said to be serving as a
discriminative stimulus (or cue). A wide variety of discriminative
stimuli are encountered in everyday life, ranging from those imposed
arbitrarily (e.g. traffic lights) to the naturally occurring (body
language!).

It should be no great surprise that common laboratory animals can
exhibit remarkable expertise in using environmental events as discriminative stimuli, provided that the stimuli are in a modality for
which the subject possesses the necessary sensory apparatus. Thus,
rats are exceptionally capable in tasks requiring the detection of taste
stimuli, while pigeons have extraordinary visual abilities and can
respond even to the dimming of light transmission produced by
microscope slide cover-slips (paper-thin, clear glass). What may be a
surprise (it certainly was for pharmacologists) is that animals can be
extremely capable at detecting the presence in their bodies of a wide
range of psychoactive drugs. Indeed, under suitable conditions, such
'drug discrimination' behaviour can develop at least as quickly as
behaviour involving the discrimination of conventional external
stimuli, and the final degree of stimulus control can be very marked
indeed. Schuster and Balster (1977) provide a general review of the
topic.

The ability of drugs to serve as discriminative stimuli became
known largely through the pioneering work of Overton in the 1960s,
mainly using maze-running techniques. Other workers soon adapted
the conventional apparatus of operant conditioning (the 'Skinner
box') to the task. In some early experiments of this type, the drug was

applied in a manner functionally equivalent to the use of the external tone stimulus in the example given above; pressing a bar was reinforced only in sessions preceded by administration of a drug. For example, food reinforcers might be delivered on a fixed-ratio schedule in sessions beginning fifteen minutes after injection of the central nervous system stimulant, amphetamine; in sessions after injections of physiological saline (control solution), bar pressing would have no consequences.

After exposure to a sufficient number of such drug and non-drug training sessions given in random order, rats immediately start to bar-press after injections of amphetamine, but withhold responding in its absence. Amphetamine may therefore be producing stimulus control in a manner functionally equivalent to the audible tone in the earlier example; the main difference is that the source of the stimulus is internal istead of external. However, this particular procedure (the one-bar, 'go or no-go' task) is now little used. The measurement of stimulus control is in terms of response rates and most drugs have marked direct, unconditioned effects on response rates; these effects are very easily confounded with changes in stimulus control.

The most common procedure is now the two-bar discrimination task, the introduction of which is generally credited to Barry and his associates. The subject is presented with two response bars. For half of the subjects in an experiment, pressing the bar on the left side of the test chamber is reinforced in sessions following drug injections, whereas pressing the bar on the right side of the chamber is reinforced after injections of physiological saline. Responses on the wrong bar are neither reinforced nor punished. For the other half of the subjects, these side-drug relationships are reversed to balance out the effects of any natural preferences for responding on one or the other bar. In this situation, drug-produced stimulus control is assessed by indices of *which* bar the subject 'chooses' to respond on, rather than simply by response rates.

It is vitally important to ensure that other cues are not confounded with drug effects; for example, once a reinforcer has been obtained in a given session, the subject could use its delivery as a cue for correct responding throughout the rest of that session. There are several ways around this problem; one method involves the use of special test sessions, called extinction tests, where no responses are reinforced. These tests are interspersed between the regular training sessions. The degree of drug-produced stimulus control may be expressed as the percentage of the total number of responses made on the drug-appropriate bar (e.g. 100 × left bar responses/left bar responses + right bar responses, for subjects trained to respond on the left bar after drug injections).

Behaviour in this type of situation has now been studied in several species, with a number of response topographies (bar pressing, tube licking, key pecking, etc.), and with a variety of schedules of reinforcement. Generally speaking, the ease with which drugs acquire stimulus control over behaviour is not much influenced by schedule variables (such as the nature of the reinforcer or the use of ratio, interval or other schedules). The type and dose of drug are the most important variables; if the dose used is too small, then only weak stimulus control develops. If the dose is too large, the behaviourally toxic effects of the drug will suppress all responding and training will be impossible. However, with appropriate doses of many widely used psychoactive drugs, very powerful stimulus control develops within thirty to forty training sessions. In such cases, after saline injection, less than 10 per cent of the total number of responses during a five-minute extinction test will be on the drug-appropriate bar; after drug injection the percentage of drug-appropriate responding may reach 90 per cent or more.

During these extinction tests, it is only the ability of the subject to detect the effects of the drug in its body which determines the bar upon which responses are made; there is no correlation with changes in response rates produced by the drug, or with changes in perception of external stimuli due to the drug. The latter possibility has been excluded by various experiments, including local applications of drugs to sensory organs.

Once a subject has been trained with a given drug, a number of further investigations can be undertaken. These often include varying the dose of the drug or giving doses of some other substance. Figure 3.1 shows some typical results in rats trained to discriminate the effects of cocaine, a powerful central nervous system stimulant. There is a clear relationship between the dose of cocaine and the percentage of drug-appropriate responses. Figure 3.1 also shows what happens when amphetamine is substituted for cocaine in the same subjects; amphetamine produces a dose-related increase in the percentage of drug-appropriate responding and in adequate doses, the effect is equivalent to that of the training dose of cocaine. These results are in the form of dose-response curves which are also psychophysical

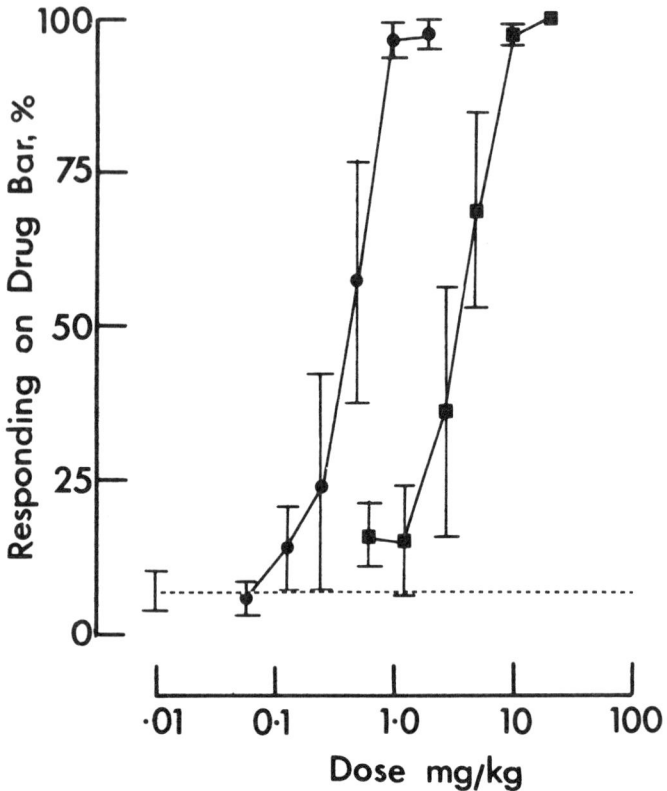

Fig. 3.1 Dose-response curves for amphetamine (●) and cocaine (■) obtained from five rats trained to discriminate cocaine (10 mg/kg) from saline. The horizontal dashed line shows the low level of drug-appropriate responding after saline; the strong degree of drug-produced stimulus control can be seen from the switch of responding to the drug-appropriate bar after suitable doses of either amphetamine or cocaine. All data were obtained during five-minute extinction tests and vertical bars show one standard error each side of the mean.

Source: Stolerman and D'Mello (1981a).

generalization gradients; the subjects indicate how they perceive stimuli (drug doses) which differ from the training stimuli. Thus amphetamine produces the same type of stimulus as cocaine and is 'generalized' with it. However, amphetamine produced this effect at doses only about one-fifth of the size of the cocaine doses, as shown by the shift to the left of the dose-response curve for amphetamine. This fits in with the known high potency of amphetamine in other tasks. The position of such dose-response curves is also much influenced by the dose used for training; the lower the training dose, the lower the doses of drugs which can be detected subsequently in generalization tests. The qualitative nature of the drug-produced stimuli also changes to some extent as the training dose is varied. Drugs which differ substantially from the one used for training often do not increase drug-appropriate responding above the saline control scores, and the implications of this will be considered below.

Applications of drug discrimination behaviour

The class in which a drug is perceived as belonging greatly influences the uses to which it is put. The usual classification for psychoactive drugs is based on a mishmash of their chemical structure, major pharmacological effects (in experimental situations) and clinical uses (see Chapter 1). The results of behavioural tests contribute importantly to such classifications, and drug discrimination methods are being used increasingly often for this purpose.

Once an animal has been trained to discriminate the effects of one particular drug from the non-drug condition, it is often the case that only drugs of the same pharmacological class are generalized with it. For example, consider rats trained to discriminate amphetamine; when other drugs are administered in generalization tests, only those compounds with central stimulant actions like those of amphetamine increase drug-appropriate responding. If depressant drugs such as barbiturates, pain relievers such as morphine, or hallucinogens are given, drug-appropriate responding does not increase; instead the rats continue to press the saline-appropriate bar. The trained rats can thus be used as a 'litmus-paper' for amphetamine-like activity.

Equivalent work has been done with subjects trained to discriminate representative central nervous system depressants and opiates and with compounds of many other classes. By and large, the classification of drugs according to the similarity or otherwise of their discriminative effects correlates very well indeed with the traditional classification (Barry, 1974).

Drug discrimination behaviour, therefore, offers the possibility of a standard technology for the classification of drugs with widely differing actions which normally have to be studied with very diverse procedures.

The results are objective and quantitative in the sense that the relative potencies of different drugs can be compared. Like every other pharmacological test that has ever been devised, discrepancies can occur, and 'false' positive or negative results may sometimes be obtained from generalization tests. One major limitation seems to be with the drugs regarded as hallucinogenic in humans; many of these compounds are readily discriminated by rats or monkeys, but sometimes they are generalized with drugs which are not hallucinogenic. For example, quipazine is generalized with lysergic acid diethylamide (LSD) in rats but it is not hallucinogenic in humans. Whether there really are species differences is not certain; formal discrimination experiments with these drugs have not been carried out in humans. It is also possible that LSD does not produce hallucinations in animals housed in the common, rather barren, laboratory environment, and that the LSD discriminative stimulus is based on some other action of the drug.

The considerable degree of pharmacological specificity shown by many drug-produced stimuli is itself somewhat surprising; intuitively, one might expect that when a subject receives a drug different from both the training stimuli (drug and saline), it would respond randomly on both bars until a reinforcer was obtained. As in other areas of behavioural pharmacology, intuition is a bad guide to what actually happens; such subjects very often emit the response appropriate for the non-drug condition. One interpretation of this finding is that the discrimination acquired is not between normal and abnormal states, but is between the presence and absence of the very specific effects of a particular drug, regardless of whether other 'abnormal' drug-produced stimuli are present.

A second area in which drug-discrimination techniques are used is in the analysis of the neurochemical mode of action of drugs. Pharmacologists are very much concerned with how drugs interact with chemicals naturally present in the brain, since the behavioural effects of drugs are thought to be mediated through them. Many such brain chemicals are called neurotransmitters because their release in minute quantities provides the crucial link whereby one nerve cell communicates with another. Different neurotransmitters act at very different receptor sites. Administered drugs may act to mimic the action of the natural neurotransmitter substance by activating the same receptor sites, or by occupying these sites without activating them; in the latter case, the normal action of the transmitter is blocked. Other drugs may act by stimulating the synthesis or release of neurotransmitters, or by interfering with the processes which normally inactivate the transmitter after it has done its work at the receptor site. Researchers both in academia and the pharmaceutical industry sometimes use drug discrimination techniques as behavioural assays in such work (Rosecrans and Glennon, 1979).

The usual way to proceed is to compare the effects of the drug under study with reference compounds whose neurochemical effects are known from previous work. Apomorphine in low doses selectively activates receptor sites upon which the neurotransmitter dopamine acts. Rats trained to discriminate the effects of cocaine or amphetamine show drug-appropriate responding when given apomorphine in generalization tests (Figure 3.2). P-hydroxyamphetamine has peripheral effects similar to those of amphetamine, but does not penetrate easily into the central nervous system; this drug does not produce discriminative effects like those of cocaine or amphetamine. Drugs such as haloperidol, used clinically to treat schizophrenia, are known to selectively block dopamine receptor sites when given in small doses; these drugs have also been found to block the discriminative stimulus effects of amphetamine or cocaine when administered shortly before responses to the latter compounds are tested. Such results support the view that the discriminative stimulus properties of cocaine and amphetamine involve actions at central nervous system receptor sites that are normally targets for the neurotransmitter dopamine.

The drug α-methyl-p-tyrosine (AMPT) prevents the synthesis of dopamine and pretreatment with this substance blocks the discriminative effects of amphetamine. This suggests that intact tissue stores of dopamine are essential for amphetamine's actions, which are thought to be mediated indirectly through the release of stored dopamine. AMPT does not block responses to apomorphine, which acts directly on dopamine receptors, or to cocaine which, although very similar to amphetamine in many ways, seems to act through a slightly different mechanism. Two-bar drug discrimination techniques are particularly suited to such work just because the responses assessed are discriminative in nature; selective effects of drugs can be distinguished from the non-specific depression of all behaviour which can make experiments on, for example, locomotor activity so difficult to interpret. The main disadvantage is the considerable time, skill and expense involved in training animals, which can make testing

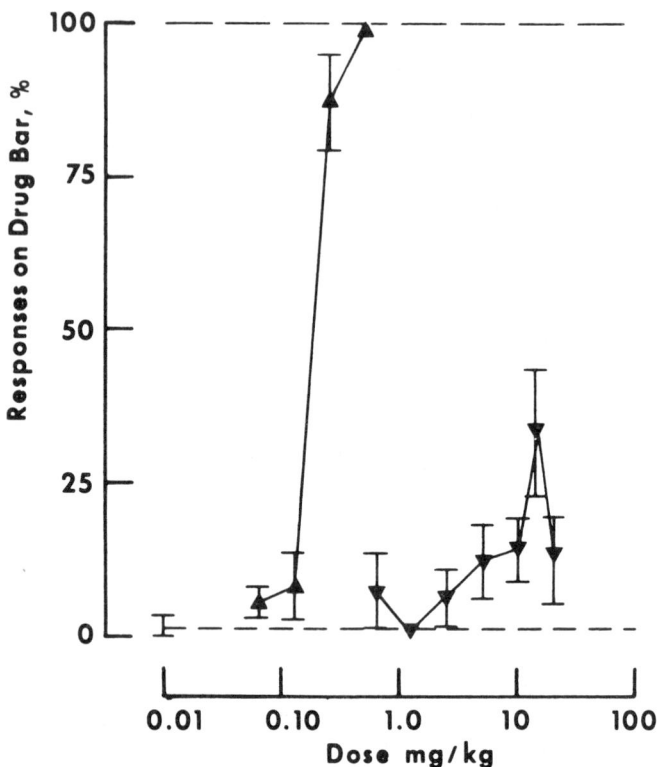

Fig. 3.2   Dose-response curves for apomorphine (▲) and *p*-hydroxyamphet-amine (▼) in five rats trained to discriminate cocaine (10 mg/kg) from saline. The horizontal dashed lines show stimulus control produced by 10 mg/kg of cocaine (— — —) or saline (– – –). Thus, the rats generalized apomorphine but not *p*-hydroxyamphetamine with cocaine.

Source: Stolerman and D'Mello (1981a).

large numbers of drugs expensive and long-winded. This means that the potential for applications of the technique is mainly at the later stages of drug development and that its use in the initial screening of new compounds is likely to remain rather limited.

Psychological significance of drug-produced cues

In the preceding sections, drug-produced stimulus control was discussed operationally; what it looks like and what it can be used for were outlined. Little consideration was given to which effects of the drugs formed the basis for the cues, or to whether drug cues were related to other known psychological effects of the agents concerned.

On the whole, it seems as if drug discrimination behaviour can be understood in terms of much the same conditioning principles that apply to the discrimination of conventional external cues. It appears to be the major psychological effects of drugs that are discriminated, rather than side-effects. Drugs within the traditional pharmacological classes have major effects in common but their numerous other actions (side-effects) vary considerably; if side-effects were the basis of most drug discriminations, it would not be possible to obtain consistent cross-generalization only between drugs in the same class. Most drug-produced cues emanate from the central nervous system; this further supports the view that it is psychological effects which are detected, yet the precise nature of these effects remains elusive. It is very likely that many drugs are discriminated on the basis of several related effects (a 'stimulus complex'), but it is very difficult to identify which effects when there are no clearly defined sensory organs involved, as there are with external stimuli.

Psychoactive drugs, almost by definition, produce changes in subjective state, feelings and mood in humans. Such effects have been extensively studied by standardized methods under controlled conditions. In this way it is possible to determine whether a novel drug produces subjective effects similar to a reference substance, for example the narcotic analgesic drug morphine.

In tests with large numbers of drugs, there has emerged a remarkable correlation between reports of morphine-like (predominantly euphoriant) subjective effects in former narcotic addicts and the results of generalization tests in animal subjects trained to discriminate the effects of morphine. Only those narcotic analgesic drugs which produce morphine-like effects in humans produce discriminative effects identified by rats or monkeys as morphine-like. Such positive results were obtained with many very addictive narcotic drugs such as heroin, methadone and fentanyl. Less addictive analgesic drugs, and compounds from other pharmacological classes (aspirin, hallucinogens, central nervous system stimulants and depressants) are not identified by animals as producing morphine-like discriminative stimuli. Thus the properties of morphine which enable it to function as a discriminative stimulus in animals seem analogous to those responsible for producing subjective effects in humans.

This type of observation is exciting because at first sight there is at last a means for assessing in animals something approximating to mood in humans. Paradoxically, drug discrimination experiments seem to make it possible to assess subjective effects objectively; perhaps something is wrong here. Correlational evidence is notoriously difficult to interpret reliably in terms of cause and effect. Just what is a 'subjective effect' in a human? Perhaps subjective effects are manifestations of the discriminative stimulus properties of drugs, rather than the other way about.

Schuster and his associates (1981) have examined the processes involved in measuring drug-produced subjective states from a behavioural point of view. Subjective states are assessed either from pencil-and-paper inventories of mood changes or from verbal self-reports. Instructions to the subjects indicate that they should respond in the manner which best reflects how they feel at that moment. The responses before and after drug are compared with responses to placebos (dummy pills or injections) to determine whether the drug has produced a significant change. It has often been assumed that the self-reports accurately represent matching between the subjects' feelings and the statements made, but there is no way to check this.

The self-reporting can be viewed as operant behaviour controlled by its consequences, and thus sensitive to a variety of environmental influences. Powerful control over verbal behaviour can be exerted by subtle responses of the experimenter, while the subjects remain unaware that this is happening. The existence of such influences raises doubts about the accuracy with which mood changes are reported. The suggestion has been made that such conditioning influences may have a critical role in the development of 'self-report behaviour'.

Children may be differentially reinforced for correctly labelling colours, sounds and other external events. In an analogous manner, they may be differentially reinforced for verbal behaviour considered by others to accurately describe their subjective state. The child who says she is sad when crying after a favourite toy has been broken is reinforced; if she smiles and presents a good school report, she is reinforced for saying she is happy (Schuster *et al.*, 1981). Thus, adults may have remarkably similar conditioning histories, with different verbal behaviours associated with different internal states. When these internal states are produced or altered by drugs, appropriate discriminative, verbal behaviour may occur. The subjects whose self-reports on drug effects are studied may in effect be performing a discriminative task not so very different from that performed by animals in drug discrimination experiments. The so-called 'subjective effects' of the drugs may be the result of a natural history of conditioning which has close parallels with the conditioning history of the animal subjects. Thus, conditioning history rather than purely pharmacological or inherited species characteristics may be a major determinant of the correlation between the findings in humans and animals.

State-dependent learning is a phenomenon which is closely related to drug discrimination. Behaviour originally acquired under the influence of a drug is not always fully exhibited in the absence of the drug, and vice versa. Such behaviour is said to be 'state-dependent' since it is disrupted either by the *change* from the drugged to the non-drugged state, or from the non-drugged to the drugged state, rather than by the direct effects of the drug itself. There is an analogy with non-drug contextual (background) cues where a learned response is only fully manifested in the presence of environmental stimuli present when it was acquired. State-dependency may sometimes be a problem when drugs are used in conjunction with psychotherapy or behaviour modification techniques, and may also be produced by alcohol and nicotine. In laboratory situations, state-dependency is measured by increased response latencies, lower response rates or more errors. Continuing research with human and animal subjects is necessary for its full significance to become apparent.

Drugs as motivating stimuli

Positive reinforcing effects

An environmental event which increases the frequency of responses with which it is associated is called a reinforcing stimulus or reinforcer. When the situation is such that a specified response leads to the administration of a drug, the ability of the drug to serve as a positive reinforcer can be tested. An increase in the frequency of the response thus results in the development of drug-taking (self-administration) behaviour. Drugs, like conventional external stimuli, are said to have the ability to *serve as* reinforcers rather than to be reinforcers since such effects are not invariant and immutable but are dependent on various antecedent and current circumstances.

The earliest systematic studies suggesting that drugs might be able to serve as reinforcers were carried out by Nichols in the 1950s. Solutions of morphine were made available to rats as an alternative to their usual drinking water, and it was eventually possible to demonstrate progressive increases in the consumption of the morphine solutions. Later workers further developed this approach to the extent that rats consumed about twice as much morphine solution as plain water, despite its very bitter taste. Equally bitter but pharmacologically inactive solutions of quinine were not consumed under these conditions. The idea that the rats consumed the morphine for its pharmacological effects was further supported when it was demonstrated that injections of morphine shortly before morphine/water choice tests selectively reduce drug intake in a dose-related manner, without suppressing the overall fluid intake (Kumar and Stolerman, 1973).

These experiments on the oral intake of morphine were interpreted within the context of operant conditioning and certainly suggested that the drug might serve as a reinforcer, but there was no clearly defined operant response involved and it was difficult to carry out the usual schedule manipulations. The next step was the application of conventional operant conditioning methods in conjunction with techniques for automatically delivering drug injections under the control of automatic equipment. By 1961, Weeks had connected rats with fine tubes (catheters) permanently implanted in their jugular veins to motor-driven syringe pumps. If bar-presses were followed by injections of morphine through the catheter, the rate of bar-pressing increased and the animals administered substantial amounts of morphine to themselves. This technique eliminated problems due to the taste of the drug and the delay of reinforcement which complicated work with the oral techniques, and greatly facilitated the use of well-defined operant responses and intermittent schedules of reinforcement. Similar results with monkeys were soon obtained by Thompson and Schuster and the hunt was on for other drugs which might also have reinforcing effects.

The next major development was in 1968, when Pickens and Thompson reported that rats would bar-press to obtain infusions of the psychomotor stimulants, amphetamine and cocaine. Figure 3.3 shows samples of some control experiments carried out to test whether the apparent positive reinforcing effects were due to unconditioned, response-rate increasing effects of the drugs. It can be seen that bar-pressing was maintained only if the rat had to respond in order to receive cocaine and not if the same doses of the drug were given 'free' (Figure 3.3A), or if the drug infusion were terminated (Figure 3.3B and C). The rat also 'tracked' the drug if infusions could only be obtained by switching responses from one bar to another (Figure 3D). Similar findings were soon obtained in other laboratories and intravenous drug self-administration was subjected to intensive study (Johanson, 1978).

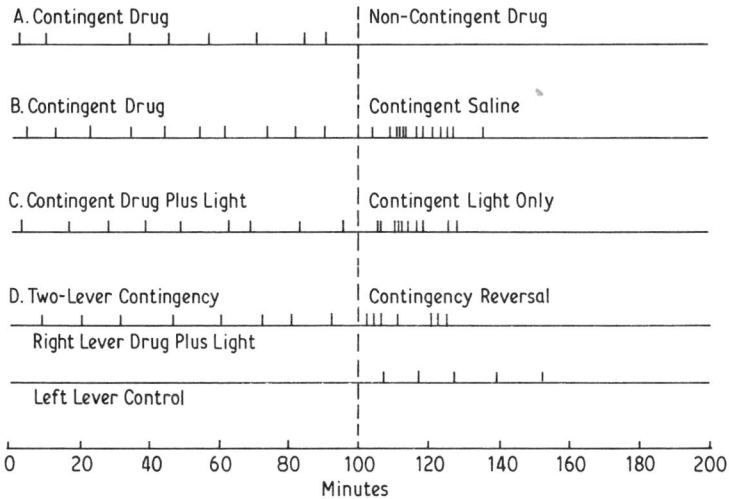

Fig. 3.3 Effects of varying relationship between bar-press responses and intravenous infusions of cocaine (0.5 mg/kg) in rat with implanted venous catheter. Responses are shown as vertical deflections on records. Changes in contingencies relating responses to injections of cocaine were made at the dashed, vertical line, 100 minutes into each session.

Source: Pickens and Thompson (1968).

It is known that if the amounts of amphetamine or cocaine given in each infusion are varied, then the animals adjust their response rates in such a way as to obtain approximately constant hourly doses of the drugs. It is also possible to maintain responding on intermittent schedules of reinforcement. Figure 3.4 shows records of behaviour from squirrel monkeys responding under fixed-interval and fixed-ratio schedules of cocaine reinforcement. During the fixed-ratio schedule, high overall response rates are maintained; during the fixed-interval schedule overall response rates are lower and a characteristic 'scalloped'

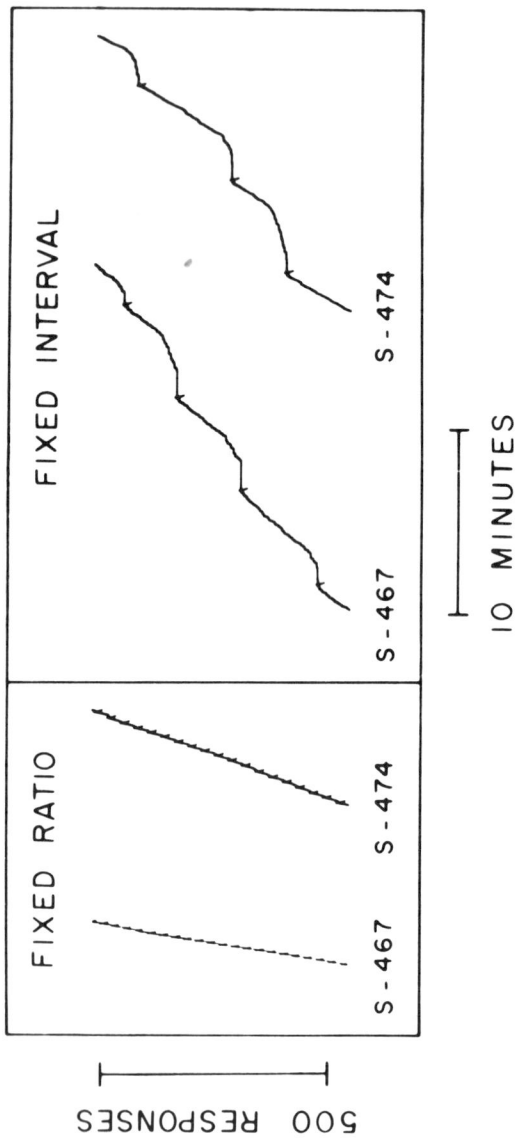

Fig. 3.4 Cumulative records showing performances under fixed-ratio or fixed-interval schedules of intravenous cocaine injection in two monkeys (S-467 and S-474). Vertical axes show cumulative number of responses. Horizontal axes show time. Left segment shows samples of records from sessions in which a thirty-response fixed-ratio schedule was in effect. Right segment shows samples from sessions in which a five-minute fixed interval schedule was in effect. Each short diagonal stroke on the records indicates an intravenous infusion of 25 µg/kg of cocaine.

Source: Goldberg *et al.* (1975).

pattern of responding is obvious. Thus, the behaviour maintained by schedules of cocaine reinforcement shows some of the main characteristics of behaviour maintained by schedules using conventional reinforcers. When the number of responses required under the fixed-ratio schedule is varied, animals alter their overall response rates so as to maintain approximately constant numbers of cocaine infusions per session.

The patterns of drug-taking behaviour which are derived from studies of the positive reinforcing effects of drugs have been of great interest as an animal analogue of drug addiction in humans. The contribution of this approach to an understanding of addiction is considered below. It is necessary to realize that simply showing that an animal will self-administer a drug is not equivalent to showing that the drug can serve as a pharmacological reinforcer. For example, a great number of experiments on alcohol drinking in rodents are virtually uninterpretable due to the transient nature of the behaviour or inadequate control for taste factors. Drug-produced reinforcement is demonstrated only by an increased frequency of responding when drug self-administration is the sole consequence of the response. Obvious signs of intoxication from the self-administered drug are neither necessary nor sufficient for it to be defined as a reinforcer.

Aversive effects of drugs

Possible aversive effects of stimuli can be assessed by either punishment or negative reinforcement procedures. A stimulus is defined as a punisher when it decreases the frequency of a response with which it is associated. For example, an electric shock or a blast of air in the face may decrease response rates if presented when a bar is pressed to obtain food.

In morphine-dependent monkeys, intravenous infusions of the narcotic antagonist naloxone appear to act as punishing stimuli. Dependence in these animals is maintained by injecting morphine several times a day; when such injections are stopped or naloxone is given, the morphine-withdrawal illness is produced. The apparent punishing effect of naloxone may be mediated through the withdrawal reaction that it produces However, in morphine-dependent subjects, naloxone can suppress responding either when given in a response-contingent or non-contingent manner. Thus, the apparent punishing effect is very difficult to separate from a general, unconditioned response-rate decreasing effect. This common problem considerably complicates the use of the punishment paradigm in assessing the stimulus effects of drugs, and probably accounts for the limited use it has had to date.

A stimulus is defined as having negative reinforcing effects when behaviour which is associated with its *termination* increases in frequency. Bar pressing may occur more often when it terminates an electric shock or a stimulus that signals shock (escape and avoidance behaviours). Goldberg and colleagues have shown that morphine-dependent monkeys can learn to press bars to terminate infusions of naloxone. Such experiments can demonstrate very clearly whether a drug serves as a negative reinforcer; the effect sought cannot be confounded with the ubiquitous response-rate decreasing effects of drugs since negative reinforcement is shown by increases in response rates.

Another procedure which has often been considered to test for aversive effects of drugs is called conditioned taste aversion (CTA). These methods have come into prominence mainly through Garcia's work, and some unusual characteristics of the effect have implications for behavioural pharmacology as well as for theories of learning (Revusky and Garcia, 1970; Domjan, 1980).

In the typical CTA experiment, the subjects are allowed to consume a distinctively flavoured but harmless fluid (or food); shortly after access to the solution is stopped, a drug is injected. The subjects are then allowed a reasonable period, usually a few days, to recover from the direct effects of the drug, and are then retested for consumption of the distinctively flavoured solution. A reduced intake of the solution is considered as evidence for the conditioning of 'taste aversion' and hence, the drug is regarded as having an aversive effect according to this criterion.

Two remarkable aspects of CTA seem to defy conventional ideas about what can be learned. Firstly, powerful conditioning can be obtained with long time delays between presentation of the conditioned stimulus (tasty solution) and the unconditioned stimulus (drug effect). Reliable conditioning with delays of several minutes is commonplace and even periods of several hours can be tolerated (albeit with rather weaker CTA as the result). The phenomena traditionally studied by learning theorists are not usually resistant to delays of more than seconds, sometimes fractions of seconds. The dependence of CTA on the nature of the stimuli used is also unusual.

In rodents, only weak conditioning is obtained if auditory or visual stimuli are used in place of the taste cues, although these stimuli can be readily associated with the effects of electric shock. It is also very difficult to produce CTA with shock, the most widely studied aversive stimulus in conventional experiments. These relationships are highly species-specific and have promised to provide an account of how learning abilities match to the ecology of different species. However, there is now considerable doubt as to whether the ability to support CTA indicates that a drug has aversive effects in the usual sense of the term, as used in studies of punishment and negative reinforcement. The difficulty arises mainly because no correlation has been found between the ability of drugs to produce CTA and their aversive effects in the other paradigms (Stolerman and D'Mello, 1981b).

Lithium and apomorphine were the drugs most frequently used in earlier studies of CTA. Both of these substances are known to produce nausea and vomiting in humans and it was assumed that some type of toxic effect, gastro-intestinal distress or nausea, was the basis for CTA in rats. Naloxone is also potent and very effective in producing CTA in morphine-dependent subjects; however, merely because a drug such as naloxone supports both CTA and operant escape/avoidance behaviour, it does not follow that it is serving a similar stimulus function in both cases.

As long ago as 1971, Cappell and his co-workers had shown that CTA could be produced by many psychoactive drugs that had not previously been thought to have aversive effects. The list of such drugs has been considerably extended and now includes amphetamine, barbiturates, alcohol and morphine. Figure 3.5 illustrates the typical CTA produced by amphetamine. Far from being merely toxic or emetic, such agents are actually capable of supporting operant self-administration behaviour by serving as positive reinforcers. These observations have stimulated much work on a so-called 'paradox'; how can the same agent both serve as a positive reinforcer and yet have aversive properties?

Common preconceptions about the determinants of behaviour frequently delay acceptance of unexpected research findings such as the potency of addictive drugs in CTA: however, there are ample precedents establishing that the same event can serve either positively reinforcing or aversive functions. This seems to be the case both with common external stimuli such as electric shock and with narcotic antagonist drugs. There should be little more difficulty in accepting

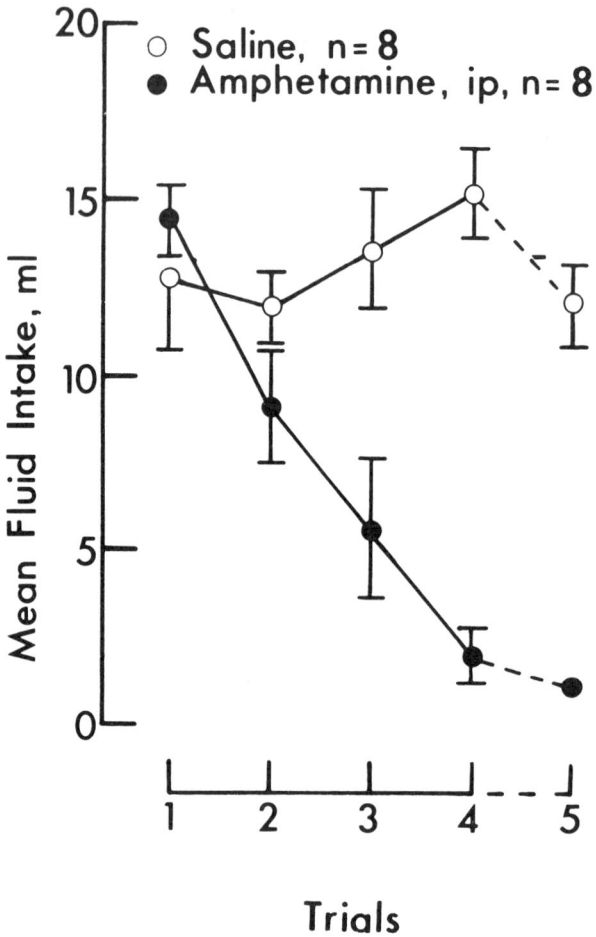

Fig. 3.5   Conditioned taste aversion produced by (+)-amphetamine (1 mg/kg) in rats (n = 8). In fifteen-minute test sessions, the mean consumption of flavoured solutions fell progressively when each period of access to them was followed by injection of amphetamine (● : trials 1—4). The consumption of control flavoured solutions remained relatively constant when saline was injected (○). On trial 5, development of CTA was confirmed in a test where both amphetamine-paired and control flavoured solutions were presented simultaneously. Direct effects of amphetamine on fluid intake do not influence these results since the drug was always injected *after* the period of drinking.

Source: Stolerman and D'Mello (1981b).

that, for example, amphetamine can serve superficially contrasting stimulus functions than in accepting that it can either increase or decrease the rate at which behaviour is emitted according to dose, schedule-associated factors or the previous history of the organism. All drugs have multiple unconditioned effects and can probably serve multiple stimulus functions (for a review, see Stolerman and D'Mello, 1981b). Nevertheless, CTA does not provide a straightforward way of testing possible aversive effects of drugs, in either the everyday sense of the term aversive, or in the empirical sense in which it is used in operant conditioning research.

Drug addiction

The non-medical uses of drugs and the development of drug dependence continue to excite controversy. The traditional pharmacological approach has emphasized the effects of repeated or long-term administration of drugs, such as the development of tolerance and the drug withdrawal illness (abstinence syndrome). Acquired tolerance to the effects sought by users was regarded as associated with progressive increases in the doses taken, which in turn exacerbated the intensity of the withdrawal reaction. Prevention of the unpleasant withdrawal syndrome was seen as a major motive for the continuation of drug use. The difficulty was that tolerance and dependence were primarily *consequences* of prolonged use, rather than initiating factors. Not all drugs produced withdrawal reactions and, sometimes, even those drugs known to produce withdrawal were taken so infrequently and in such small doses as to make very unlikely the occurrence of the withdrawal syndrome. It is also known that both human and animal subjects self-administering alcohol allow themselves to go into repeated periods of withdrawal, despite the availability of alcohol all the time.

Psychiatrists, on the other hand, have often sought to explain dependence in terms of abnormalities in individual psychology and personality, and have emphasized a role for an inadequate ability to cope with stress. These accounts tend to assume that there is an addiction-prone personality, but this has not yet been identified except perhaps in highly selected populations. Explanations are often offered in terms of 'craving' to take drugs, but such factors cannot be assessed independently of the behaviour they purport to explain. It is important not to underestimate the contributions that the traditional approaches have made, although actual drug-taking behaviour was not developed and analysed under controlled experimental conditions. The application of the ideas and methods from experimental psychology, especially operant and classical conditioning techniques, have considerably enhanced knowledge of variables which can control drug-taking behaviour. Such work also shows ways in which the pharmacological processes (tolerance and withdrawal syndromes) can be influenced by conditioning. Many of these ideas were embodied in theoretical articles which have been extant for decades, but their practical realization was dependent on recent technological advances and has taken a long time.

The fundamental datum of the behavioural approach to dependence has been the demonstration that addictive drugs can serve as unconditioned positive reinforcers. In suitable circumstances, animals will self-administer most of the drugs that produce dependence in man, and such self-administration is maintained by the positive reinforcing effects of the drugs. The compounds taken in this way include the psychomotor stimulants, narcotic analgesic drugs, barbiturates, benzodiazepine tranquillizers, alcohol, nicotine, and volatile solvents (used by 'glue sniffers'). Many psychoactive drugs not associated with dependence in man are not reinforcing in animal tests; these include some appetite suppressants, antidepressants, neuroleptics, narcotic antagonists and some drugs with a mixture of narcotic and narcotic antagonist effects. The major discrepancy lies with the hallucinogenic compounds and cannabis (including its active constituents); these substances are generally not found to serve as positive reinforcers in animal tests.

It is remarkable that the reinforcing effects of drugs are manifested in laboratory animals without the need to produce any underlying 'emotional' dysfunction through either genetic or environmental manipulations. The drugs are taken in the absence of any attempt to induce 'animal models' of psychopathology by, for example, adverse environmental or other stressful conditions. A previous history of drug-produced tolerance and withdrawal reactions is also unnecessary for drugs to serve as reinforcers. Drug-naïve animals can be trained to self-administer morphine and then stable patterns of responding can be maintained over long periods of time (month after month), despite the doses taken being too small to produce detectable withdrawal effects. Animals can also relapse rapidly to drug taking after long periods of enforced abstinence, in some cases a year in length. A limited amount of recent work has also shown that addictive drugs can serve as reinforcers in humans, although for ethical reasons these studies have involved only known drug users.

An important line of work on the role of secondary reinforcement in drug dependence has developed from the more fundamental studies of drugs as primary reinforcers. Secondary (conditioned) reinforcers are environmental stimuli which have acquired reinforcing effects through their association with primary (unconditioned) reinforcers. Thus a red light may be turned on for five seconds whenever a subject self-administers morphine. After a sufficient number of red light-morphine pairings, the red light alone can greatly increase the number of infusions taken when saline is substituted for morphine. This finding suggests that the red light has acquired reinforcing effects through association with morphine, and it is an interesting example of the influence of a classical conditioning process on operant behaviour.

In the example given above, the red light maintains responding for only a limited amount of time since its effects are soon extinguished in the continued absence of the primary reinforcer, morphine. However, it is possible to construct a 'second-order' schedule of reinforcement in which responding is maintained by brief environmental stimuli which are occasionally paired with a primary reinforcer (Goldberg *et al.*, 1975). For example, the self-administration of cocaine has been studied in monkeys under a schedule where the completion of each thirty-response fixed ratio produces only a two-second yellow light until five minutes have elapsed; the first fixed ratio completed after five minutes produces both the yellow light and an intravenous infusion of cocaine. Monkeys maintained on this schedule respond at very high rates for prolonged periods of time. Yellow lights alone do not maintain responding and overall response rates for cocaine in the absence of yellow lights are relatively low in the conditions used. Thus, stimuli which are occasionally associated with the infusion of reinforcing drugs can themselves maintain responding, probably because they acquire secondary reinforcing effects.

In other experiments involving second-order schedules, subjects have responded at steady, high rates for hours on end, with the only consequence of responding being the presentation of brief visual stimuli; at the very end of the sessions, these brief stimuli are paired with injections of the primary reinforcing drug. These experiments show how secondary reinforcers can maintain responding during long periods when the drug itself is not available, and have obvious implications for understanding the persistence of drug-seeking behaviour in humans. In the search for methods to help people stop taking drugs, it is necessary to take account of the possible effects of secondary reinforcers; such conditioned effects may occur even when the primary reinforcing effects of the drug itself have been blocked pharmacologically (perhaps with a narcotic antagonist such as naloxone or naltrexone).

Although drugs can maintain self-administration behaviour by serving as reinforcers, it does not follow that such effects are the sole determinants of the amounts taken. The self-administered drugs may have direct, unconditioned effects on response rates, and this means that simple rate measures may be unreliable indicators of a drug's potential for producing dependence.

Considerable efforts have been made to develop more satisfactory means for quantifying a drug's reinforcing efficacy. One method involves the use of progressive ratio schedules; within a session there is a gradual increase in the number of responses required to obtain the drug reinforcer. The highest ratio of responses to reinforcers which maintains behaviour provides the measure of reinforcing strength in the progressive ratio procedure. Another approach allows the subject a choice between a standard drug dose and a different dose of the same drug (or a different drug altogether). In such tests, monkeys generally self-administer the larger of two doses offered, even if this dose normally has marked response-rate-decreasing effects and would not maintain much behaviour under simpler schedules of reinforcement.

Aversive effects of drugs, which might appear mainly at high doses, may also limit the amounts taken in self-administration experiments. Present knowledge makes assessment of this phenomenon difficult, and it is not known to what extent such effects actually limit drug intake in the usual experimental or practical situations where drugs are taken. Regardless of the precise conditioning mechanisms involved, conditioned taste aversion experiments indicate that very powerful behavioural suppression can be produced by many self-administered drugs. Interestingly, excessive doses of nicotine produce nausea and vomiting in human users of tobacco and probably set an upper limit to its use; in animals, nicotine is effective as a punisher of operant responses and is also very potent in producing conditioned taste aversion.

The relationship between the reinforcing and subjective effects of drugs has been the subject of much discussion. This matter is a part of the wider problem of the nature of reinforcing stimuli and associated changes in affect. It is simplistic to assume that pleasurable subjective states are necessary for stimuli to serve as reinforcers since in suitable subjects, noxious electric shocks can serve as positive reinforcers. The pleasure-pain principle seems equally inapplicable to pharmacological reinforcers. After appropriate training, morphine-dependent monkeys repeatedly self-administer naloxone. This narcotic antagonist then precipitates the morphine withdrawal reaction which is very unpleasant for humans and makes the monkeys look very ill. Many other drugs may be self-administered at very high doses which produce obvious signs of toxicity, which may include convulsions, coma or self-mutilation. It is hard to believe that these are pleasurable effects, yet the drugs which produce them are undoubtedly serving as reinforcers. Furthermore, in long-term studies on humans, some drugs continue to function as reinforcers despite the development of dysphoric (unpleasant) effects; other drugs continue to produce euphoria but do not continue to serve as reinforcers.

Conclusions

The preceding text should have made it abundantly clear that drugs can serve as stimuli in a great variety of conditioning situations. All the major stimulus functions identified in earlier research can be fulfilled by drugs, and the extent of conditioning developed to drugs is often equivalent to that developed to traditional external stimuli. This chapter has concentrated on the motivational and discriminative stimulus effects of drugs, but the same substances can be programmed to serve as the unconditioned stimuli in classical conditioning procedures. This opens a wide field for consideration since, in addition to the traditional Pavlovian experiments involving responses of the autonomic nervous system, interactions with operant behaviour become very pertinent; here there are many instances where previously neutral stimuli become conditioned to drug effects and can themselves modify response rates, serve as reinforcers, etc. A complete understanding of the behavioural effects of drugs has to take into account these diverse stimulus properties.

The practical applications which have been most prominent to date have been in aspects of new drug development and classification, in studies of the neurochemical mechanisms of drug action, and in the

82   Aspects of Psychopharmacology

behavioural analysis of some specific problems, such as drug dependence. Perhaps the field will also make some contribution to an understanding of the nature of subjective states and their relations with behaviour, although some new element may need to be introduced for much further progress to be made here. The future should also reveal whether neurotransmitters and hormones naturally released in the body during the normal course of its functioning actually bring about some of their effects by serving as stimuli which control conditioned responses.

References

Barry, H., III (1974) Classification of drugs according to their discriminable effects in rats. *Federation Proceedings 33*: 1814–24.

Domjan, M. (1980) Ingestional aversion learning: unique and general processes. *Advances in the Study of Behavior 3*: 275–336.

Goldberg, S. R., Kelleher, R. T. and Morse, W. H. (1975) Second-order schedules of drug injection. *Federation Proceedings 34*: 1771–6.

Johanson, C. E. (1978) Drugs as reinforcers. In D. E. Blackman and D. J. Sanger (eds) *Contemporary Research in Behavioral Pharmacology*. New York: Plenum, pp. 325–90.

Kumar, R. and Stolerman, I. P. (1973) Morphine dependent behaviour in rats: some clinical implications. *Psychological Medicine 3*: 225–37.

Pickens, R. and Thompson, T. (1968) Cocaine-reinforced behavior in rats: effects of reinforcement magnitude and fixed-ratio size. *Journal of Pharmacology and Experimental Therapeutics 161*: 122–9.

Revusky, S. and Garcia, J. (1970) Learned associations over long delays. In G. H. Bower (ed.) *The Psychology of Learning and Motivation: Advances in Research and Theory*. New York: Academic Press, pp. 1–84.

Rosecrans, C. R. and Glennon, R. A. (1979) Drug-induced cues in studying mechanisms of drug action. *Neuropharmacology 18*: 981–9.

Schuster, C. R. and Balster, R. L. (1977) The discriminative stimulus properties of drugs. In T. Thompson and P. B. Dews (eds) *Advances in Behavioral Pharmacology*. Vol. 1. New York: Academic Press, 85–138.

Schuster, C. R., Fischman, M. W. and Johanson, C. E. (1981) Internal stimulus control and the subjective effects of drugs. In *Behavioral Pharmacology of Human Drug Dependence*. National Institute on Drug Abuse Monograph 37. Washington, DC: US Government Printing Office, pp. 116–29.

Stolerman, I. P. and D'Mello, G. D. (1981a) Role of training conditions in discrimination of central nervous system stimulants by rats. *Psychopharmacology 73*: 295–303.

Stolerman, I. P. and D'Mello, G. D. (1981b) Oral self-administration and the relevance of conditional taste aversions. In T. Thompson, P. B. Dews and W. A. McKim (eds) *Advances in Behavioral Pharmacology*. Vol. 3. New York: Academic Press, pp. 169–214.

4 Alcohol and alcoholism

Geoff Lowe

'It is helpful, at the risk of
oversimplification, to consider the effects
of alcohol in four stages — dizzy and
delightful, drunk and disorderly, dead
drunk, and dead.'
(Office of Health Economics)

Introduction

All that is necessary to manufacture alcohol is to permit a sweetened
liquid, such as berry juice, to stand in a container in a warm place for
a few days. Consequently, nearly all cultures have early discovered the
effects of alcoholic beverages roughly simultaneously with their
development of simple containers that could hold liquids. The
remarkable, almost universal, phenomenon is that each culture
making these discoveries also found such pleasures in sampling the
results that there soon developed the abuse of alcohol.

There is little doubt that alcohol affects our behaviour in a multi-
plicity of ways . . . and apparently has done for ages. In the past,
alcohol research has been something of a scientific stepchild, rel-
egated to breweries and a few pharmacologists interested in its anaesthetic properties; and for the most part the research was ephemeral
and casual. But in recent years a growing number of basic scientists
have been attracted to the subject. In the field of psychopharmacology, researchers have found the effects of alcohol a useful tool in

the study of fundamental psychological mechanisms, while others have been interested in such research for clinical reasons. Consequently the psychopharmacology of alcohol as a research area is expanding rapidly in breadth and depth. Certainly the experimental investigation of alcohol's effect on the central nervous system and behaviour, and of the dependence process produced by the drug, has achieved a reasonable measure of scientific respectability. Alcohol research centres are rapidly gathering momentum and a new science of 'intoxicology' is about to emerge.

Perhaps the greatest proliferation in this area has been in animal research (see Meisch, 1977; Myers, 1978), where controlled experiments enable systematic assessment to be made of variables uncontaminated by the usual complex interplay of influencing factors in the human psychosocial environment. However, this chapter is concerned mainly with the effects of alcohol on human behaviour, and only brief reference to animal studies will be made, where they have particular relevance to our understanding of some of the psychobiological mechanisms involved in the use and abuse of alcohol.

Alcohol intoxication

General effects and blood-alcohol concentration

Alcohol is a depressant agent, capable of impairing, retarding and disorganizing the functions of the central nervous system (CNS). Nevertheless, many of the overt behavioural effects of alcohol are stimulant. The behaviourally arousing effects of alcohol are partly attributable to a general tendency for CNS inhibitory processes to be more susceptible to disruption than are the excitatory processes. A further contribution to the behavioural stimulation caused by alcohol is a compensatory response, counteracting the depressant drug effect.

Alcohol is often classified with the barbiturates as a sedative/ hypnotic. These drugs have in common a marked depressant effect on behaviour, indicated by stupor or anaesthesia, at doses only slightly higher than 'arousing' doses.

Table 4.1 indicates typical effects at different levels of blood-alcohol concentration (BAC). Peak BACs usually occur during the span of 30 to 60 minutes after fairly rapid drinking of a given quantity of alcohol.

Table 4.1

BAC (mg/100 ml)	Psychological/clinical effects*	Time for all alcohol to leave body (hrs:mins)
20	Negligible	1:20
30	Possible slight flushing and a little more talkative than usual	2:00
50	Relaxation, lowering of inhibitions in non-tolerant drinkers. Impaired attention, impaired vigilance	3:20
60–99	(a) Impaired sensory function Reduced visual activity (flicker fusion test) Decreased sense of smell and taste Elevated threshold for pain (b) Motor inco-ordination Spontaneous and induced nystagmus Decreased steadiness when standing Impaired psychomotor performance (c) Changes in mood and behaviour Dizziness Reduced sense of fatigue Mild euphoria Self-satisfaction Louder, profuse speech (d) Impaired mental activity	4–6 hrs
100	Significant feelings of intoxication More failures in sensorimotor tracking Staggering when blindfolded More errors in arithmetical calculations Impaired short-term memory	6:40
150	Staggering when eyes are open Lengthened reaction time Marked impairment on mental and psychomotor tests Slurred speech	10:00

Table 4.1—continued

BAC (mg/100 ml)	Psychological/clinical effects*	Time for all alcohol to leave body (hrs:mins)
200	Responsiveness to stimuli abolished Extreme clumsiness Nausea and vomiting	13:20
250	Marked tendency to pass out	16:40
300	Hypothermia Amnesia Anaesthesia Slow, heavy breathing	20:00
400	Comatose	26:40
500	Breathing abolished Death	—

* These approximations are given for determinations obtained during the ascending limb of the BAC curve. During this period the mental effects are more pronounced and the mood tends to be more euphoric. On the other hand, as BAC declines, at equivalent levels the mental effects are less pronounced, and more negative feeling tones are experienced.

These figures are approximations and do not take into account a sex difference in body fat. Since females have 10−20 per cent more body fat, which excludes most of the ethanol, the same ethanol intake in terms of body weight (g/kg) results in higher BAC in females than in males. Thus, the same quantity of alcohol consumption by a typical woman results in appreciably higher BAC not only because of her lower body weight but also because of her higher proportion of body fat.

A standard drink is defined as either 12 oz of beer, 5 oz of dry wine or $1\frac{1}{2}$ oz of 80° proof spirits. These quantities contain approximately the same amount of alcohol. Alcoholic beverages between 4 and 44 per cent provide similar BACs. Below that percentage the alcohol absorption may be delayed by the large fluid volume. Above that percentage pylorospasm may delay absorption.

About 90 per cent of alcohol consumed is metabolized by liver-produced enzymes, particularly alcohol dehydrogenase. The rate of oxidation is fairly uniform for each person averaging 15 mg/100 ml (0.015 per cent) per hour with a range of 0.012 to 0.018 per cent. This is equivalent to the metabolism of 1 g of pure alcohol for every 10 kg of body weight per hour.

The rate of destruction of alcohol is independent of the BAC except at levels above 0.3 per cent (300 mg/100 ml) when other enzymes like catalase and the microsomal endoplasmic oxidizing system of the liver come into play. The remaining 10 per cent of the ingested alcohol is excreted virtually unchanged by the lungs and kidneys with small amounts eliminated by the skin. It is difficult to accelerate the metabolism of alcohol. The time course of elimination can be shortened by up to 20 per cent by eating fructose, but the amounts needed are large and would probably cause stomach cramps. However, physical, stressful exercise may increase metabolism rate somewhat. This is possibly brought about via breath and sweat excretion.

Although intestinal fermentation produces up to an ounce of ethanol a day, the alcohol dehydrogenase system is efficient enough to degrade it immediately. Therefore a person who has consumed no alcohol in beverage, medicinal or food forms will have a zero BAC. Rare individuals, however, with inefficient systems, can have permanently raised BACs.

Since the rate of removal of alcohol from the blood is fairly constant, it is unnecessary to obtain a breath or blood sample immediately following an event. By retrospective interpolation over the time elapsed between the event and the actual sample, a corrected reading should approximate the BAC at the specified event time. Alcohol remaining in the stomach at the time of BAC testing could lead to error in such calculations: therefore BAC samples should not be obtained until 20 minutes have elapsed since the last drink.

The BAC or blood-alcohol level (BAL) is a reliable and reproducible measurement of ethanol in the blood. Since alcohol diffuses uniformly to all tissues, it is also a reflection of brain ethanol levels. Breath alcohol determinations are more frequently used for practical purposes and converted by a factor of about 2300 so that the apparatus automatically provides a BAC reading.

Three different ways of reporting BAC are used, and this may lead to occasional confusion. Table 4.2 gives examples of each for the BAC which is the present legal limit (in Britain).

Although the BAC is quite reliable, the variance is about ± 10 per cent. Thus, two tests are preferable to a single determination. The test is

Table 4.2

G/100 ml (%)	Mg/100 ml (mg/dl)	G/litre (promille)
0.08	80	0.8

not a measure of the amount of ethanol consumed. Body weight is especially important, and rapidity of drinking, time elapsed since last drink, the particular ability of the drinker to metabolize alcohol, the presence of food in the gastro-intestinal tract and other factors will determine the BAC. For example, a man weighing 85 kg (187 lbs) consuming 4 pints of beer in 1 hour would ingest 3.2 oz (91 g) of ethanol. His ethanol consumption would thus be at a rate of 1.07 g/kg/hr, resulting in a BAC of approximately 107 mg/100 ml (0.107 per cent). A woman, weighing 55 kg (121 lbs) consuming a 12 oz can of lager/beer and 3 'shorts' in an hour would be ingesting 2.3 oz (65 g) of ethanol. Her ethanol consumption would be at a rate of 1.18 g/kg/hr, resulting in a BAC of approximately 118 mg/100 ml (0.118 per cent).

Subjective reports of intoxication are important because they provide our closest access to the subjective cues that govern drinking behaviour in a single drinking session. Ekman *et al.* (1964) and others have found that such ratings can be made with some degree of meaning. However, it is clear from other studies that the meaning or intensity of subjective intoxication varies greatly according to dose level and alcohol habits. Although there is an overall relationship between BAC and subjective ratings (SR) as a function of time, the correlation is much greater over the ascending limb of the BAC curve. As BAC decreases the disparity between BAC and SR becomes more marked, with SR declining faster (see Figure 4.1).

Banks *et al.* (1979) have suggested that our alcohol 'sensor' processes a host of sensory and proprioceptive cues and is therefore subject to sensory adaptation effects. They argue that perception of the present state of intoxication is a function of both the present and previous levels of blood alcohol. Thus, a given BAC may lead to a high subjective rating if the preceding levels were lower, and a low subjective rating if the preceding levels were higher. Rising BACs are more subjectively intoxicating than falling BACs.

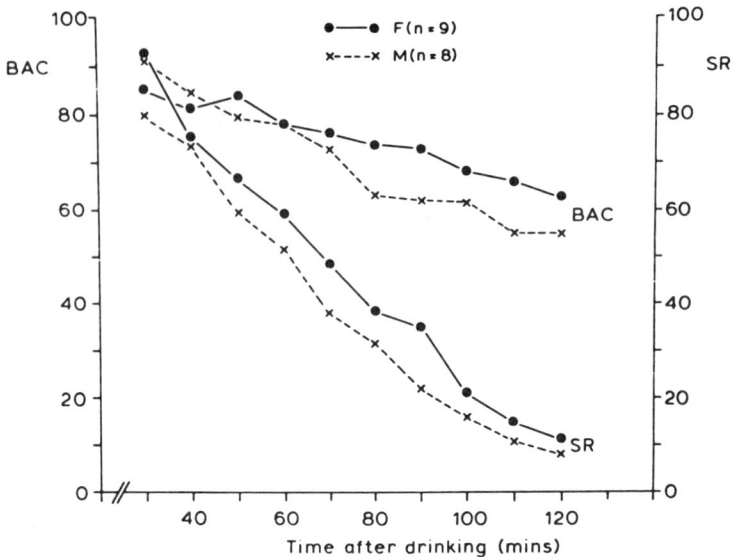

Fig. 4.1   Relationship between blood-alcohol concentration (BAC), subjective rating (SR) of intoxication, and time after drinking in males and females. SR values refer to distances, in cms, of a mark drawn by the subject on a horizontal scale line ranging from 'absolutely sober' to 'very intoxicated'.

Effects on human performance

There is little doubt that alcohol can affect various aspects of human performance. But when we ask more precise questions about which kinds of task, under what conditions, and under what dosages, then several features of the alcohol literature cause difficulty in any attempt at generalization or integration (Levine *et al.*, 1975). Some of these factors include: differences in type of control conditions (e.g. repeated measures versus independent group designs); differences in subject population (e.g. sex, weight, age and type of drinker); differences in methods of alcohol administration (fixed dose per person or mg/kg body weight); differences in type of alcohol (e.g. different alcoholic beverages have different rates of absorption); variations in time allowed to consume alcohol, time of day, and time between ingestion and testing (there are important differences in effects due to ascending and descending blood-alcohol concentrations (Jones and Jones, 1976); wide range of tasks with various dependent and independent variables.

In general, cognitive and perceptual-sensory performances are most disrupted by alcohol; psychomotor tasks seem to be more resistant, although measurable decrements can still be observed. Moskowitz (1979) has reported the sensitivity of attention, perception and information processing to moderate and even low doses of alcohol and other drugs. Since these are the areas of crucial importance for skills performance in complex man-machine interaction situations, such findings suggest why activities such as driving are so susceptible to alcohol-induced disruption.

There is considerable evidence that alcohol intoxication interferes with memory and learning processes. The most severe memory disturbance is the alcoholic 'blackout', an inability to recall events that happened during a drinking episode, even though consciousness was neither significantly clouded nor lost. A decreased ability to recall may take place at blood-alcohol levels of 40 mg/dl, and it seems to progress in a linear fashion as the level rises.

One of the major difficulties in determining and explaining these memory deficits is that the effects of acute intoxication wear off after a few hours, leaving the person in a different physiological state. What is learned under a drug state (i.e. while drunk) is not so well recalled when tested under a sober state (and vice versa). Retention is, however, greater when the original drug state is reinstated (Lowe, 1981). State-dependent learning is the term used to describe this phenomenon. Such 'dissociation' of learning between drunk and sober states has led to the speculation that state-dependent learning may be a factor in the aetiology of alcoholism and may at least partly explain memory loss for events occurring while drinking. Even drinking immediately *after* sober learning may affect consolidation with resultant recall deficits if there is drug-state dissociation between storage and retrieval phases (Lowe, 1982).

Alcohol, expectancy and stress

The relationship between alcohol and stress has long been a concern in the alcohol research literature. Various studies have primarily focused on determining whether a stressful situation increases the amount of alcohol consumed. Positive findings have been interpreted in terms of subjective anticipation of alcohol's effectiveness in dealing with stress; this implies some type of cognitive mediation as an explanation for the drinking response. Recent evidence has shown that many of the behavioural effects of alcohol are, in fact, largely due to covert expectancy factors, and a 'balanced placebo' design has been suggested by Marlatt and Rohsenow (1980), to differentiate psychological and physiological factors in any alcohol experience.

The 'tension reduction hypothesis' is a model for relating alcohol and stress that has generated much controversy (e.g. Cappell and Herman, 1972). The hypothesis proposes a drive reduction model, which requires that the organism be in some high-drive state (e.g. tension or anxiety) and emit the response of consuming alcohol. This response is then reinforced by means of its ability to reduce the drive state. The model has not been easy to test, however, and experimental paradigms have differed in the way stressful states have been introduced. Additionally, special problems are incurred when 'tension' is operationally defined by different physiological measures. However, in a recent, well-designed study, Levenson *et al.* (1980) derived clear indication that alcohol consumption is associated with reduction in the magnitude of response to stress. Specifically, they found attenuation of the magnitude of response to two kinds of stressors (self-disclosing speech and threat of shock) in both physiological and psychological measures. This 'stress response dampening' is consistent with the notion that alcohol has a positive value when consumed in the context of a stressful situation.

Another approach which has been applied to this problem is to manipulate the subject's affective state prior to ad-lib drinking situations. Clearly, if alcohol is used to alleviate depressive affect and anxiety, then inducing such states should stimulate drinking behaviour. Pihl and Yankofsky (1979) assigned subjects to one of two conditions designed to induce either positive (incentive gain) or negative (incentive loss) affective states. Contrary to expectation, their analysis revealed that more alcohol was consumed by subjects in the incentive gain condition. A second analysis demonstrated that significantly less alcohol was consumed by subjects who, prior to ad-lib drinking, evinced greater degrees of depressive affect and anxiety. These results suggest that while affect can act as a potent mediator of alcohol consumption in social drinkers, the relationship is the converse of what has been commonly believed. The findings certainly contradict the tension reduction hypothesis that a palliation of negative affects provides the major form of reinforcement from, and source of motivation for, alcohol consumption.

On the other hand, it has been suggested that alcohol *per se* only serves to induce a non-specific state of physiological arousal (plasticity) which is then defined according to the cognitive context. Russell and Mehrabian (1975), for example, consider that a person's pre-consumption affective state and the setting where drinking occurs determine the cognitive context and, consequently, the affective and reinforcing value of different dosages of alcohol. Clearly, an interactionist position, emphasizing the person and the situation as well as the drug, is needed before significant progress in understanding and controlling the effects of alcohol can be made.

Modification of alcohol's effects

Subjective and behavioural effects of alcohol may vary according to the individual's state – psychological or psychological – and these modifiers may act additively, synergistically, antagonistically or in other ways. The most dramatic psychological determinants of alcohol intoxication are the sudden 'sobering effects' induced by acute fear or trauma (e.g. Barry, 1973). Various experimental studies (reviewed by Wallgren and Barry, 1970) show that physical and psychological stressors, such as pain, cold, exhaustion and conflict, may modify the actions of alcohol. Wilkinson and Colquhoun (1968) studied interactions between alcohol and sleep deprivation in their effects on a five-choice reaction time task. When subjects were classified as to BAC above or below 0.032 per cent, the low BAC group showed that thirty hours' sleep deprivation reduced the adverse effect of alcohol on performance speed whereas the high BAC group showed the opposite effect. More recently, Peeke et al. (1980), in their study of the combined effects of alcohol and sleep deprivation (twenty-six hours), found antagonism for most measures (reaction time, heart rate, alertness, anxiety) but synergistic effects also occurred.

As for the mechanism underlying the compensatory response during alcohol intoxication, it has been proposed that the adrenal hormones might play a crucial role in evoking the physiological arousal needed to counteract the depressant effects of alcohol. One hypothesis suggest that people who have an efficient adrenocortical response to stress ('stress-capable' individuals) would be less influenced by alcohol than others with weaker adrenocortical reactions. Myrsten et al. (1979) found opposite effects of a combination of alcohol and reward on psychological functions and additive effects on physiological functions. The outcome of this complex interplay was that the combined action of alcohol and reward (in an achievement situation) produced, at the same time, the highest physiological arousal level and the most favourable overall psychological response. Other studies have demonstrated that alcohol induces a general 'plasticity' which may be converted by a particular cognitive context or setting into various affective experiences and expressions. For instance, Young and Pihl (1980) asked social drinkers 'to try to stay sober' after drinking alcohol in an experimental setting. These subjects demonstrated better memory and hand co-ordination than did social drinkers who were not similarly motivated but had comparable BACs. On the other hand, Maisto *et al.* (1981), in a study of affect/sensation, cognitive and perceptual-motor performance, found their subjects could exert very little control over motor task performance while under the influence of a low (0.025 per cent) or moderate (0.05 per cent) dose of alcohol. The data did, however, indicate that low-dose subjects inaccurately perceived that they were able to counteract alcohol's effects when instructed to do so. Such inconsistencies in the available literature may stem from variations in motivation manipulation and differential expectations of the subjects.

Drug interactions with alcohol

Various centrally active drugs are assumed or known to interact with ethanol at the receptor level. With low doses of drugs and alcohol the interaction problems are often connected with driving and related psychomotor skills, whereas with larger doses poorly understood lethal interactions are encountered. The increasing use of tranquillizing agents has directed the interest of researchers on to problems concerned with the effects of alcohol when taken in combination with such drugs as meprobamate, chlordiazepoxide and diazepam. Some reports indicate that chlordiazepoxide significantly reduces some alcohol-induced effects, while diazepam enhances such effects. Meprobamate also enhances alcohol impairment. Many medicines and other social drugs may compound alcohol effects in unpredictable ways and this calls for further research to reveal important side-effects.

Alcohol is often consumed in close temporal proximity with caffeine. It is a fairly common belief that coffee will antagonize the intoxicating effects of alcoholic beverages, and it has been assumed that this antagonistic effect is due to the CNS stimulant properties of caffeine *per se*. As yet, however, there has been no evidence to support this notion. Experiments on human subjects have indicated a failure of caffeine (and d-amphetamine) to antagonize the depressant effects of alcohol. More recently, in a study of five-choice, serial reaction time, we found a significant alcohol-caffeine interaction which indicated that caffeine is capable of potentiating (rather than antagonizing) the disruptive effects of alcohol (Lee and Lowe, 1980). Moreover, this effect appears to be independent of prevailing BACs. This potentiation is consistent with the early findings of Pilcher (1911), who found that caffeine and alcohol interacted synergistically to increase fatality rates in cats. And among a variety of equivocal results, other workers have recognized the complexity of the alcohol-caffeine interaction. At a neurochemical level, Waldeck (1974) found a markedly increased synthesis of brain catecholamines (CA) in mice after combined treatment with caffeine and ethanol. This suggests that the interaction probably involves central CA mechanisms and has implications for the adrenocortical arousal hypothesis mentioned above.

The identification of a means of quickly and safely counteracting acute alcohol intoxication could provide a mechanism for reducing the dangers to the health and safety of the heavy drinker. We could also gain valuable insights into alcohol's mechanism of action and the adaptive processes that lead to drug dependence.

Once alcohol is administered, there are essentially two methods for reversing its central effects: (a) reducing the amount of alcohol in the brain by decreasing its absorption, altering its distribution, or enhancing its removal (pharmacokinetic antagonism); and (b) antagonizing its actions on the CNS (pharmacodynamic antagonism). A given drug (or, indeed, environmental manipulation) may act to reduce intoxication by either or both of these methods.

One plausible hypothesis predicts that drugs which block or otherwise attenuate CA systems should increase alcohol depression, whereas drugs which augment CA systems should antagonize alcohol depression. In general, attenuators of central CA function have been shown to markedly increase alcohol's depressant effects, but no clear relationship between CA increase and alcohol antagonism has yet been found.

Several reports of alcohol's interaction with central monoamines indirectly suggest that dopamine (DA) and noradrenaline (NA) may play different, perhaps opposite, roles in modulating alcohol's effects. Recent data indicate that specific DA stimulation augments rather than reduces alcohol depression. In contrast, NA stimulation appears to be antagonistic. Ewing *et al.* (1974) report that subjects with high plasma activity of DA-β-hydroxylase (the enzyme catalysing the biosynthesis of NA from DA), felt less intoxicated than subjects with the same BACs (66 mg/dl) but with low DA-β-hydroxylase activity. Although highly speculative, such findings support the notion that high NA availability may counteract or block some aspects of alcohol depression and may indicate a possible mediating mechanism for the alcohol-stress interaction mentioned above.

Since it appears that alcohol, like other general anaesthetics, does not act via a specific receptor, it is unlikely that any single agent, analogous to the opiate antagonists, will be discovered which reverses all aspects of intoxication. Ultimately, a useful antagonistic agent may require the combination of several partial antagonists selected for their abilities to counteract different aspects of alcohol intoxication.

Alcoholism

There is no single definition of alcoholism but several behavioural criteria taken together enable one to judge the severity of a drinking problem. Among these criteria are: 'loss of control' of drinking behaviour; psychological dependence upon alcohol ('needs a drink' to get anything done); loss of job(s), family or friends because of drinking; blackouts; increasing tolerance for alcohol; withdrawal symptoms upon stopping drinking (physical dependence).

The common factor in all drinking problems is the negative effect they have on the health or well-being of the drinker, and on his or her associates. Several authorities in the alcohol-abuse field have suggested these criteria for drinking problems: frequent drinking to a state of intoxication; going to work intoxicated; drunken driving; physical injury as a consequence of being intoxicated; breaking the law as a consequence of an intoxicated state; seriously misbehaving and using intoxication as an 'excuse'.

Although the popular image of the alcoholic person is the 'Skid-Row', derelict type, this group actually comprises only about 5 per cent of the total number. About 50 per cent of alcoholics are employed persons. It is estimated that 75 per cent of the adult population drink alcoholic beverages at least occasionally. Among these drinkers, approximately 6 per cent consume 'hazardous' amounts (more than 100 ml — about $3\frac{1}{2}$ oz or five 'social' drinks per day). And although only a much smaller percentage become addicted to alcohol, this nevertheless amounts to an estimated 350,000–400,000 people in Britain.

Whether or not the incidence of alcoholism corresponds to the incidence of people who drink in a given group is a question of some importance, since it is much more feasible to identify drinkers than it is to identify alcoholics, and data concerning the former are often used to discuss problems concerning the latter.

It is a well-recognized fact that, among Jews, the use of alcohol as a beverage is nearly universal, but incidence of alcoholism is extremely low. But in France drinking and alcoholism rates are both high. These and other similar observations indicate that incidence of drinking cannot be used as a reliable index of the incidence of alcoholism. However, it is important to distinguish between the drinking rate of individuals in a group and per capita consumption in the group as a whole; there is an apparently fixed relationship between consumption averages (in a given society) and alcoholism prevalence.

Types of alcoholism

The two main categories of alcoholics as defined by the Alcoholism Subcommittee of the World Health Organization are 'alcohol addicts' and 'habitual symptomatic excessive drinkers' (referred to as non-alcoholic addicts). In the opinion of Jellinek (1960), one of the original leading authorities on alcoholism, the disease concept refers only to the alcohol addict. Both types are characterized by excessive drinking that reflects underlying social or psychological problems. But alcohol addicts, after several years of excessive drinking, lose control, while non-addictive alcoholics do not. Jellinek observes that many excessive drinkers consume as much or more than addicts over a period of thirty or forty years without loss of control. This suggests to Jellinek that a superimposed process (perhaps psychological, perhaps physiological) makes the difference between prolonged excessive drinking and addiction.

In recent years the disease concept of alcoholism has gained widespread acceptance among both professionals and non-professionals. However, many do not accept this thesis because they see alcoholism differing greatly from other diseases like heart ailments and pneumonia. The disease theory, which holds that addiction is the result of a chemical imbalance, has not been proved. A more serviceable concept may be to term alcoholism as a behavioural disorder.

As with many other kinds of disorder, three different categories of factors or causes may operate in the development of alcoholism – physiological, psychological (individual/developmental) and social. Glatt (1974), in discussing addiction to alcohol and other drugs, stresses the interacting triad of the 'host' (i.e. the individual), the 'environment' and the 'agent' (i.e. the pharmacological nature of the drug concerned).

Physiological factors

The simplistic approach to alcoholism is the notion that alcohol causes alcoholism: hence, no alcohol, no alcoholism. But, as we have observed, only a small proportion of the millions of drinkers become alcoholics, hence the possibility must be considered that the physiology of some persons makes them particularly susceptible. Much effort has been exerted to find chemicals in specific beverages which might be responsible for alcohol addiction, or physiological, nutritional, metabolic or genetic defects which could explain excessive drinking.

The clearest case for the role of physiological factors in the development of alcoholism would be provided by the existence of hereditary tendencies. It is true that children of alcoholics often end up the same way. But alcoholism also occurs in those whose parents are abstainers. Moreover, children of alcoholics can be protected if they are reared away from their parents. This strengthens the belief that alcoholism is related more to environmental than to genetic factors. Nevertheless, McClearn (1973), of the Institute of Behavioral Genetics, University of Colorado, argues strongly for a model of alcoholism that includes genetic parameters. His results from selective breeding in rats and mice demonstrated that avidity for alcohol and differential sensitivity to its effects have heritable bases. The problem remains, however, of extrapolation from animals to man.

It has been suggested that alcoholism is caused by vitamin deficiencies or hormone imbalances. However, most of the nutritional and hormonal deficiencies observed in chronic alcoholics appear to be the result rather than the cause of excessive drinking.

At the present stage of research, the evidence seems to weigh against any notion that alcoholism is caused exclusively by physiological factors. That there is differential physiological sensitivity to alcohol, however, seems indicated, with the strong possibility that physiological factors may contribute to alcoholism's development. It has been noted that in the development of alcoholism, different individuals move through its sequence of stages at different rates, varying from several months to many years. It is possible that physiological factors may play some role in the differential rates.

Psychological and environmental factors

It is believed by some people that alcoholics are psychologically 'different', that they possess a number of traits which in common make up the 'alcoholic personality'. There is, however, no agreement on the identity of these traits, nor on whether they may be the causes or the results of excessive drinking. If there is an actual 'alcoholic personality' (or a 'pre-alcoholic personality'), its specifications are poorly defined and often contradictory, and seem to apply broadly to all mental illness. However, certain factors common to many alcoholics may play a part in the disorder. One of the most popular theories is that the individual drinks to remove anxiety. Intuitively this seems quite plausible, which may explain the considerable attention it has received (e.g. Hodgson *et al.*, 1979). Several experiments with animals have clearly illustrated the efficacy of alcohol in reducing fear. Some human studies have used psychophysiological indicators – basal skin conductance (BSC) which reflects chronic tension level, and galvanic skin response (GSR) which reflects reactivity to emotionally arousing stimuli. The results confirm the widespread assumption that very moderate amounts of alcohol may reduce emotional tension (see p. 92). For some highly anxious individuals, tension reduction is probably a vital factor in producing drinking behaviour. For most alcoholics, however, anxiety reduction is probably just one of several reinforcers of drinking and may not have provided the initial motivation. Further theories have been concerned with conflict over sex role, low frustration tolerance, and feelings of guilt – to mention just a few, but there is no conclusive evidence of an alcohol-prone personality.

The role of environmental factors (such as availability of alcohol, social, cultural, religious factors) in the aetiology of alcoholism has also been illustrated in a variety of studies. Of particular interest here is the notion of 'locus of control' and its relationship with alcoholism. Donovan and O'Leary (1978) found that hospitalized alcoholics having an external orientation based on 'Drinking-related Internal-External' scores were more preoccupied with alcohol, had more prolonged drinking problems, and manifested more loss of control when drinking. (More internality is correlated with better control.) In a more recent study, Jones *et al.* (1981) observed that persons reporting more perceived control over both intrapersonal and interpersonal pressures to drink (internal scorers) became reliably less intoxicated from alcohol during a 6-month period than people reporting less control (external scorers). The notion of 'locus of control' could be an especially useful explanatory concept for much of the variability found in studies of chronic alcohol consumption.

Adaptation of alcohol intoxication

As mentioned early, the ability to monitor intoxication state is subject to adaptation effects. It is possible that alcoholics may adapt to the effects of alcohol even more quickly and thoroughly than moderate drinkers do. Alcoholics sometimes report they do not 'feel' alcoholic drinks when they have quite high BACs. Increased adaptation rather than reduced overall sensitivity to alcohol may be responsible for these effects, and may also explain alcoholic 'binge' drinking. Because of adaptation, the alcoholic must drink more and more, at an accelerated rate, in order to maintain the subjective effect of alcohol. It is possible then that adaptation differences, based on reliable subjective ratings, might be used to distinguish abusers (or potential alcoholics) from normal drinkers.

Treatment of alcoholism

Obviously the treatment of alcoholism cannot be undertaken except on a pragmatic basis until the problem of causes is solved. The evidence suggests that alcoholism is a complex product of possibly physiological and certainly psychological and sociological factors. This complexity bears upon the problem of treatment, for characteristically some things work in some cases, but not in others. The best results seem to be brought about by a combination of treatments — pharmacological, psychological and social.

Pharmacological treatment

The various types of pharmacological treatment are primarily directed towards detoxification, mitigation of withdrawal symptoms, and the treatment of the deleterious physiological effects of prolonged alcohol use. Without adequate medical care for acute intoxication and severe withdrawal symptoms, the patient may not survive. Until recently, alcohol substitutes such as chloral hydrate and paraldehyde were used to mitigate withdrawal symptoms; but today's tranquillizers, together with the control of fluid and electrolytic balance, permit most patients to recover from delirium, hallucinations, and tremors relatively quickly.

While detoxification and treatment of the conditions resulting from prolonged alcohol use do not, of course, cure alcoholism, they are often necessary preliminary steps for such treatment. Once detoxification and the mitigation or partial reversal of chronic disorders are accomplished, however, drug therapy is frequently employed to start the patient on the road towards control of his actual alcoholism.

Inasmuch as tensions and anxieties often trigger drinking, tranquillizing drugs seemed to be a logical substitute for alcohol. While they are often highly effective, the alcoholic tends rapidly to become addicted to them, exchanging one form of dependence for another that may be worse in the long run.

That tranquillizers reduce tension appears to be well authenticated, but a consequent reduction in drinking does not necessarily follow. In fact, several studies, using chlordiazepoxide, have reported that in the post-withdrawal state this drug significantly reduced anxiety and increased the feeling of well-being in alcoholics while, paradoxically, increasing the tendency to drink. A possible explanation of this is that the increased sense of well-being and self-confidence may mislead the patients into believing that they can easily handle alcohol, or perhaps that they have no drinking problem at all.

Antipsychotic and antidepressant drugs are typically of little, if any, value in the treatment of chronic alcoholism. Nevertheless, a survey of psychiatrists in the USA found alcoholism to be the third most frequent disorder for which psychotropic drugs were prescribed, with schizophrenia and depression ranking first and second respectively. It is distressing (but not too surprising) to find such widespread use of psychotropic drugs in a condition for which the efficacy of drug treatment remains largely unproven.

Another basically pharmacological approach which has been more commonly used is deterrent therapy, using drugs which sensitize the body to alcohol, such as disulfiram (Antabuse). Alcoholics are given these in tablet form in hospital for a few days and then they are given a sample of their usual brand of alcohol. Ten minutes or so after drinking (just sufficient to produce the reminiscent smile and feeling of well-being) the patient finds that the warm glow he knows so well is getting out of hand. He then begins to suffer extremely distressing symptoms – severe flushing, eyes becoming distended and bloodshot, sweating, nausea, breathlessness and feeling like dying. If unduly distressing, the effects can be promptly terminated by counteracting drugs.

The effects of Antabuse occur only if a patient takes alcohol within about three days of taking a tablet. Thus the treatment plan calls for one tablet to be taken daily. Although this requires a certain amount of determination on the part of the alcoholic, it is advantageous in that he need only take one decision a day – to take the tablet – rather than the many involved in resisting the urge to drink. Thus Antabuse is a 'chemical fence' around the alcoholic, forcing him to be abstinent and supplying time for other therapies to be attempted (Faiman, 1979).

It is more than possible that drugs similar to Antabuse may set a limit upon how much an alcoholic can slip back into drinking. A study of alcoholism in Japan, for instance, describes a cyanamide compound that allows a patient to drink about 8 oz of wine per day before an unpleasant reaction sets in. If too much is drunk, sickness results. The idea is that after a few experiences the patient should conclude that his illness results from excessive drinking and should moderate his intake accordingly.

These drugs act as conscious deterrents against drinking, provided, of course, that the alcoholic has become fully convinced of the possible consequences of drinking during the treatment regime and is fully co-operative in taking the tablets. Because of the complex aetiology of alcoholism, many alcoholics are characteristically nowhere near this level of co-operativeness.

Psychological treatment

Alcoholism is not an illness in the usual sense, but may be more of an ineffective and inappropriate means of managing emotions and frustrations — a coping mechanism that masks rather than eliminates the real sources of difficulty. Because the roots of the problems or difficulties are (generally) neglected, there is always the possibility that they may, in fact, be aggravated. In this sense, alcoholism constitutes a maladaptive approach to life and it requires more 'treatment' than the simple removal of the inappropriate coping technique — alcohol use.

Recent psychological approaches consider alcoholism as constituting a complex behaviour pattern and thus theoretically amenable to various methods of behavioural control. Psychotherapy is a general label for a wide variety of procedures which attack the problem of alcoholism at the level of the individual's conscious and emotional experience. Trained professionals seek to raise the level of the individual's insight into his own problems, while at the same time giving whatever counselling and guidance will help to bring drinking under control. When psychotherapy is successful, it is presumably because of a transformation of attitude and emotion on the part of the patient that renders drinking behaviour irrelevant.

The systematic use of behaviour modification and treatments based upon social learning formulations offers a promising new alternative to traditional methods. Within this framework alcohol abuse is seen as a learned behaviour pattern (socially acquired), and shaped and maintained by reinforcement contingencies. However, the shaping and control of behaviour is not necessarily the same as learning new patterns. Thus a comprehensive behavioural model requires a twofold approach to treatment — firstly, techniques which suppress excessive drinking by decreasing the immediate reinforcing properties of alcohol, and secondly, techniques specifically designed to encourage non-drinking behaviour or behaviour incompatible with alcohol abuse.

The notion that chronic alcoholics can learn to drink in moderation is a new and highly controversial one. Total abstinence has been the emphatic goal of traditional alcoholism treatment. However, some proponents of behaviour modification are attempting treatment based on supervised controlled drinking practice. Indeed, recent clinical evidence suggests that some chronic alcoholics can return to and maintain social drinking patterns (Heather and Robertson, 1981; Sobell and Sobell, 1973). Such methods might be especially appropriate in the case of 'loss-of-control' alcoholics.

One point which may be relevant to the notion of controlled drinking is the likely incidence of alcoholism in the offspring of alcoholic parents. Since the children of both alcoholic and strictly abstemious parents (i.e. those with extreme views) are more likely to become alcoholic than children of more moderate parents, it would eventually be worthwhile to determine the extent of this risk in the children of 'controlled', as opposed to 'abstinent', formerly alcoholic parents.

An ingenious way to produce moderate drinking patterns involves training patients to discriminate their own blood-alcohol levels (Lansky *et al.*, 1978). Through periodic feedback while drinking, patients are trained initially to discriminate the behavioural effects which typically accompany various blood-alcohol levels, and asked to estimate their own levels. Electric shock is then made contingent upon concentrations exceeding some criterion level (typically 0.065 per cent). Some success has been achieved with some patients, but the results can only be regarded as tentative at this stage. The discrimination of blood-alcohol levels is not a universal phenomenon, and normal social drinkers usually need considerable training. Since alcoholics are more experienced drinkers, they are probably more 'tuned in' to the bodily and emotional changes due to alcohol. Moreover, some alcoholics will be more 'tuned in' than others. Nevertheless, there is no consistent evidence for the notion that alcoholics differ from non-alcoholics in this ability (Shortt and Vogel-Sprott, 1981).

As mentioned earlier, state-dependent learning or 'dissociation' may be partially responsible for poor recall of events which take place during drinking. This could, indeed, constitute the basis for 'loss of control'. After a few drinks, the alcoholic 'forgets' the (negative) consequences of heavy drinking – consequences usually experienced in a sober state. Thus, if state-dependent learning is a prominent characteristic of alcoholic drinking, then therapy should be undertaken in both the sober and intoxicated states. By contrast, alcohol-induced consolidation failure implies that various techniques for strengthening registration and consolidation of learned information must be emphasized during therapy.

Research on these issues seems to indicate that therapy for alcoholics might well be provided during periods of both sobriety and intoxication, in a combined effort to maximize consolidation and retrieval capability. Ways in which this could be done might include: (1) over-learning (which is apparently incompatible with state-dependent learning effects) during the initial registration phase; (2) using cueing devices for prompting recall of originally learned behaviour; (3) using short-term memory tasks to predict subsequent longer-term recall (further training might be necessary if short-term memory impairment is indicated); (4) monitoring blood-alcohol level carefully, so that therapy can be given during falling blood-alcohol level when drinkers are more resistant to cognitive impairment than during rising blood-alcohol level; (5) assessing the blood-alcohol level or drug-state discriminative ability of subjects, since state-dependent learning effects are more likely in more clearly discriminable drug states.

Two theories have been put forward suggesting that discriminability may indirectly cause (or be related to) alcohol dependence. One theory proposes that an altered repertoire of drug-state responses develops with repeated drug use. If the alcohol-specific behaviours are more reinforcing than normal undrugged behaviours, then the subject may use alcohol to gain access to the alcohol-response repertoire rather than because of any intrinsically reinforcing drug effects. For instance, other people may treat an intoxicated person differently (and possibly more favourably) from when he is sober. Or intoxication may alter the user's sensitivity to social reinforcement so that reinforcement contingencies are effectively changed even in the absence of any real change in the external environment.

Conclusions

The study of alcohol and its effects has become an increasingly complicated research area, its complexity being augmented by multifarious techniques and levels of analysis. A sustained effort towards improved scientific methodology would help to consolidate our understanding of basic phenomena. For instance, in view of the evidence for a biphasic effect of alcohol on the CNS, subsequent research needs to pay more attention to the time course of alcohol effects and to the dose-response relationship.

To search for the site of action or *the* mechanism of action of alcohol on the CNS seems to reflect an over-simple view of the actions of alcohol. At different degrees of alcohol intoxication, the subjective experience and behavioural manifestations may reflect different interactions of a variety of effects. Even supposing that a complete understanding of the acute effects of alcohol on the CNS suddenly emerged, our understanding of the phenomenology of alcohol intoxication would remain only partial, due to other important human determinants – predominantly 'expectancy' effects. Recent observations on the role of such cognitive factors have important methodological implications for alcohol research.

As far as alcoholism is concerned, the problems are no less complex. Many studies of alcoholics have not specified the criteria upon which a diagnosis of alcoholism was made. Even when two studies can be matched in terms of their definitions, their results may not be directly comparable if they have not controlled for age, sex, socioeconomic status, length of drinking history, pattern of drinking, types of treatment received, psychotropic medication, intelligence, neurological history, abstinence periods, etc. Not all of these will be important in every study, but some of the discrepant findings in alcoholism research might have been avoided if the population characteristics had been more clearly defined. Although considerable progress has been made (particularly in the last decade), many questions evidently remain unanswered. Is the quasi-mathematical connection between the prevalence of alcoholism and per capita consumption absolutely unalterable? What specifically determines a person's level of consumption at any point in time? What leads him to decrease or increase his consumption? What precisely are the reinforcing properties of alcohol? Why is it that only a tiny proportion of drinkers progress to hazardous levels of consumption? And why are the numbers of younger adolescent problem drinkers increasing? New solutions to these problems now seem most likely to emerge from increased emphasis on research in the behavioural, rather than the medical, sciences.

References

Banks, W. P., Vogler, R. E. and Weissbach, T. A. (1979) Adaptation of ethanol intoxication. *Bulletin of the Psychonomic Society 14*: 319–22.

Bandura, A. (1969) *Principles of Behavioural Modification*. New York: Holt, Rinehart and Winston.

Barry, H., III (1973) Motivational and cognitive effects of alcohol. *Journal of Safety Research 5*: 200–21.

Cappell, H. and Herman, C. P. (1972) Alcohol and tension reduction: a review. *Quarterly Journal of Studies in Alcohol 33*: 33–64.

Donovan, D. and O'Leary, M. (1978) The drinking-related locus of control scale: reliability, factor structure, and validity. *Journal of Studies on Alcohol 39*: 759–84.

Ekman, G., Frankenhauser, M., Goldberg, L., Hagdahl, R. and Myrsten, A.-L. (1964) Subjective and objective effects of alcohol as functions of dosage and time. *Psychopharmacologia 6*: 399–409.

Ewing, J., Rouse, B. and Mueller, R. (1974) Dopamine-β-hydroxylase and ethanol intoxication. *Research Communications in Chemical Pathology and Pharmacology 8*: 551.

Faiman, M. D. (1979) Biochemical pharmacology of disulfiram. In E. Majchrowicz and E. P. Noble (eds) *Biochemistry and Pharmacology of Ethanol*. Vol. 2. New York: Plenum.

Frankenhauser, M., Dunne, E., Bjurstrom, H. and Lundberg, U. (1974) Counteracting depressant effects of alcohol by physiological stress. *Psychopharmacologia 38*: 271–8.

Glatt, M. M. (1974) *A Guide to Addiction and Its Treatment*. Lancaster: M.T.P.

Heather, N. and Robertson, I. (1981) *Controlled Drinking*. London: Methuen.

Hodgson, R., Stockwell, T. and Rankin, H. (1979) Can alcohol reduce tension? *Behavior Research and Therapy 17*: 459–66.

Jellinek, E. M. (1960) *The Disease Concept of Alcoholism*. New Haven: Hillhouse Press.

Jones, B. M. and Jones, M. K. (1976) States of consciousness and alcohol: relationship to the blood alcohol curve, time of day, and the menstrual cycle. *Alcohol Health and Research World 1*: 10–15.

Jones, J., Coleman, G. and St Leger, S. (1981) Drinking-related control orientation and alcohol intoxication. *Psychological Reports 48*: 597–8.

Lansky, D., Nathan, P. E., Ersner-Hershfield, S. M. and Lipscomb, T. R. (1978) Blood alcohol level discrimination: pre-training monitoring accuracy of alcoholics and non-alcoholics. *Addictive Behaviors 3*: 209–14.

Lee, D. J. and Lowe, G. (1980) Interaction of alcohol and caffeine in a perceptual-motor task. *I.R.C.S. Medical Science 8*: 420.

Levenson, R. W., Sher, K. J., Grossman, L. M., Newman, J. and Newlin, D. B. (1980) Alcohol and stress response dampening: pharmacological effects, expectancy and tension reduction. *Journal of Abnormal Psychology 89*: 528–38.

Levine, J. M., Kramer, G. C., and Levine, E. N. (1975) Effects of alcohol on human performance: an integration of research findings based on an abilities classification. *Journal of Applied Psychology 60*: 285–93.

Lowe, G. (1977) Alcoholism and psychology: some recent trends and methods. In J. S. Madden, R. Walker and W. H. Kenyon (eds) *Alcoholism and Drug Dependence: A Multidisciplinary Approach*. New York: Plenum.

Lowe, G. (1981) State-dependent recall decrements with moderate doses of alcohol. *Current Psychological Research 1*: 3–8.

Lowe, G. (1982) Alcohol-induced state-dependent learning: differentiating stimulus and storage hypothesis. *Current Psychological Research 2*: 215–22.

McClearn, G. E. (1973) The genetic aspects of alcoholism. In P. G. Bourne and R. Fox (eds) *Alcoholism*. New York: Academic Press.

Maisto, S. A., Connors, G. J., Ruff, C. and Watson, D. (1981) Alcohol and volitional control on affect/sensation, cognitive and perceptual-motor measures. *Current Psychological Research 1*: 235–50.

Marlatt, G. A. and Rohsenow, D. J. (1980) Cognitive processes in alcohol use: expectancy and the balanced placebo design. *Advances in Substance Abuse 1*: 159–99.

Meisch, R. A. (1977) Ethanol self-administration: infrahuman studies. *Advances in Behavioural Pharmacology 1*: 35–84.

Mello, N. K. and Mendelson, J. H. (1971) A quantitative analysis of drinking patterns in alcoholics. *Archives of General Psychiatry 25*: 527–39.

Moskowitz, H. (1979) The effects of alcohol and other drugs on skills performance and information processing. In G. Olive (ed) *Drug-Action Modifications: Comparative Pharmacology*. Advances in Pharmacology and Therapeutics. Vol. 8, pp. 211–21.

Myers, R. D. (1978) Psychopharmacology of alcohol. *Annual Review of Toxicology 18*: 125–44.

Myrsten, A.-L., Lamble, R., Frankenhauser, M. and Lundberg, U. (1979) Interaction of alcohol and reward in an achievement situation. *Psychopharmacology 62*: 211–15.

Peeke, S. C., Callaway, E., Jones, R. T., Stone, G. C. and Doyle, J. (1980) Combined effects of alcohol and sleep deprivation in normal young adults. *Psychopharmacology 67*: 279–87.

Pihl, R. O. and Yankofsky, L. (1979) Alcohol consumption in male social drinkers as a function of situationally induced depressive effect and anxiety. *Psychopharmacology 65*: 251–7.

Pilcher, J. D. (1911) Alcohol and caffeine: a study of antagonism and synergism. *Journal of Pharmacology and Experimental Therapeutics 3*: 267–98.

Rix, J. B. (1977) *Alcohol and Alcoholism*. Montreal: Eden Press.

Russell, J. A. and Mehrabian, A. (1975) The mediating role of emotions in alcohol use. *Journal of Studies on Alcohol 36*: 1508–36.

Shortt, R. G. and Vogel-Sprott, M. D. (1981) Monitoring blood alcohol concentrations: hypotheses and implications for alcoholism. *Journal of Studies on Alcohol 42*: 350–4.

Sobell, M. B. and Sobell, L. C. (1973) Individualized behaviour therapy for alcoholics. *Behavior Therapy 4*: 49–72.

Waldeck, B. (1974) Ethanol and caffeine: a complex interaction with respect to locomotor activity and central catecholamines. *Psychopharmacologia 36*: 209–20.

Wallgren, H. and Barry, H., III (1970) *Actions of Alcohol*. Vols 1, 2. New York: Elsevier.

Wilkinson, R. T. and Colquhoun, W. P. (1968) Interaction of alcohol with incentive and sleep deprivation. *Journal of Experimental Psychology 76*: 623–9.

Young, J. A. and Pihl, R. O. (1980) Self-control of the effects of alcohol intoxication. *Journal of Studies on Alcohol 41*: 567–71.

5 Social aspects of illegal drug use

Raymond Cochrane

In many ways drug abuse is not one of the major contemporary social problems. The social consequences of illegal drug use are small when set alongside the consequences of the use of legally obtained drugs, especially alcohol and tobacco. The visible aspect of illegal drug abuse in Britain amounts to perhaps fifty to sixty deaths a year, 1500 hospital admissions, 2800 people known to be receiving narcotics on prescription because of their addiction and about 14,000 drug-related convictions. This latter figure, which swamps the others, perhaps is more properly regarded as a measure of the social reaction to drug users rather than a direct consequence of abuse. These convictions are largely for selling or possessing illegal substances and not for behaving antisocially while under their influence. Table 5.1 gives comparative figures for the known social consequences of alcohol, tobacco and illegal drug use. These figures do not reflect the other less obvious, but no less real, social costs of alcohol and tobacco use such as the cost of non-inpatient medical care, days lost from work, alcohol-related crimes, and road traffic deaths.

It must be admitted immediately that many of the figures pertaining to drug use are the proverbial 'tip of the iceberg' — few would accept that the number of addicts known to the Home Office is a true representation of the number of addicts in Britain, but inflating

Table 5.1   Estimated comparative social consequences of the use of
illegal drugs,* alcohol and tobacco per annum in Britain

	Illegal drugs	*Alcohol*	*Tobacco*
Deaths	50–60	1 800	100 000
Hospital admissions	1 500	13 500	†
'Abusers'‡	2 800	350 000	4 400 000
Related convictions	14 500	164 000	few

* Sources: Zacune and Hensman, 1971; James, 1967; Royal College of Psychiatrists, 1979.
† 5000 to 8000 hospital beds are occupied each day by people who are in hospital only because they smoke.
‡ Known addicts, alcoholics, or people smoking more than 20 cigarettes per day.

these figures by a factor of five or even ten still produces only a small
number in absolute terms. The situation is somewhat different in the
USA both because the scale of narcotic abuse is much greater even
allowing for the greater population size, and because the institutional arrangements for dealing with addictions have, in the past,
tended to exacerbate drug-related problems (such as crime) without
apparently making any significant impact on the number of drug
addicts. Even in the USA, however, drug problems are completely
overshadowed by alcohol-related problems: it has been estimated
that there might be 5.4 million alcoholics and another 20 million
Americans with serious drinking problems (Stark, 1975, p. 92). In a
stimulating paper Irwin (1973) demonstrated that the total social
and personal ramifications of the excessive eating of food in America
far outweighed the problems created by the abuse of either
marijuana or heroin.

   Why then has there been so much public concern about drug abuse
and so much energy and time devoted to studying the problem?
Firstly, it is undoubtedly true that in a small proportion of cases the
consequences to the individual of becoming a drug user can be cata-
strophic. Secondly, there have been occasions in the recent past when
it has appeared that the number of people becoming regular drug
abusers was increasing very rapidly indeed. Thirdly, and related to
the previous point, the demographic characteristics of the typical
drug user changed dramatically in the 1960s and 1970s. Previously,
drug use was believed to be confined to those in medically related

professions, because of their relative ease of access to drugs, and to very marginal social groups such as musicians, seamen and criminals. Now drug use has become established in a wider cross-section of society and is relatively more prevalent among the young. Fear of drug abuse has spread to ordinary middle- and working-class homes especially in the large cities of the USA. The increase in the number of drug addicts and the increase in the number of street crimes are also frequently associated with one another in both official utterances and in the mind of the public.

Finally, the study of the social aspects of drug abuse provides an opportunity for examining the broader category of addictive or 'excessive' behaviours. The examination of the social response to drug use also yields a fascinating insight into the social construction of a social problem.

In this chapter I will argue that an understanding of drug abuse can be gained only by considering the meaning and social context of the behaviour as defined both by the drug user and by the observer. Harré (1979), among others, has pointed out the utility of distinguishing between behaviour, action and act, and nowhere are these distinctions more valuable than in the explanation of drug abuse. There is little or no advantage in considering the mere behaviour of the drug user (or indeed, it will be argued, in considering the pharmacological properties of the drugs involved, or their effects on the user). We need to consider as well the person's intentions and goals when planning and engaging in this behaviour in order to understand the behaviour as 'action'. Ultimately, though, we will also have to be aware of the broader social meaning of the action by situating it in a social context of norms, meanings, values and beliefs. Only in this way will it be possible to begin to comprehend the reasons for, and the social response to, drug abuse.

Although not spelled out each time, the term 'illegal drug use' will be taken to refer to the non-medical use of narcotics (mainly heroin) and cannabis. 'Illegal drug use' will be used interchangeably with 'drug abuse'. 'Drug addiction' is a term usually retained for a special category of narcotic use characterized by physiological dependence and the development of tolerance. The utility of this definition is discussed in the text. Although this chapter will focus on the illegal use of two drugs (cannabis and heroin), the legal use of certain drugs as prescribed by doctors is also creating considerable concern; the examination of the social significance, in addition to the personal consequences for the patient, of the widespread and somewhat indiscriminate use of psychotropic drugs is an equally interesting topic (e.g. Cooperstock and Lennard, 1979; Koumjian, 1981; Verbrugge, 1982).

Marijuana

In a carefully controlled study of the results of marijuana smoking (often called cannabis in Britain and popularly known as pot), Weil *et al.* (1968) found that the objective effects were limited to a slight increase in heart rate, a reddening of the eyes and minimal changes in scores on performance tests (some performances got worse, some better, most stayed the same). The subjectively reported effects commonly attributed to marijuana such as euphoria, dizziness, thirst, perceptual distortions, heightened sensitivity, etc. were much more likely to be perceived by experienced users than by those using the drug for the first time. In fact several of their 'marijuana naïve' subjects could not tell whether they were actually smoking marijuana or a placebo and they could not distinguish between high and low doses. These findings have generally been confirmed by many subsequent studies. It seems that even experienced smokers of marijuana often have difficulty in distinguishing the real thing from a placebo smoked in similar conditions, although their failure to recognize anything distinctive about a marijuana cigarette is rather different from that of a naïve user. While the inexperienced smoker will have trouble in perceiving the effects of real marijuana, the more experienced user will often attribute the subjective effects of marijuana to a placebo (Galanter *et al.*, 1974; Hollister, 1971; Weil *et al.*, 1968).

This is not to suggest that cannabis contains no psychoactive chemicals – indeed in sufficient concentrations it does have very definitive hallucinogenic and intoxicating properties and acts as a mild analgesic. In general, though, these pharmacological effects can be reliably demonstrated only if the active ingredient (tetrahydrocannabinol or THC) is extracted and processed to a far higher concentration than is usually found in smoking material. According to an authoritative World Health Organization report, even long-term use of marijuana does not seem to produce any significant physical or psychological deterioration (WHO, 1972). Marijuana does not produce physical dependence, or any other medical complication, neither does tolerance develop (Stefanis *et al.*, 1977) and not a single human fatality has been attributed directly to its use (Brecher *et al.*, 1972, p. 397).

The fact that marijuana has effects which are so subtle as to appear almost negligible leads to two interesting questions. First, why has the social response to the possession and use of the drug been so massive? In several states in the USA possession of marijuana was punishable by life imprisonment, or even death, during the 1970s and there were several hundred thousand convictions a year relating to the drug (Goode, 1975). In Britain too the magnitude of the legal response seemed to far outweigh the dangers which could be attributed to marijuana use.

The second question is, simply, why do people bother to use marijuana given its minimal effects and the potential hazards if caught in possession? The remainder of this section will be devoted to answering this latter question and showing how the answers to both the questions can interact to produce an interesting social phenomenon sometimes known as 'moral panic' (Cohen, 1972).

Three, or perhaps four, stages can be identified in the development of marijuana use. Each stage can be conceived of as a filter which operates to eliminate some users but through which a decreasing proportion of others pass and become more deeply involved with the drug. These stages are initial use, regular use and 'life-style' use. Entering an environment in which marijuana is readily available is possibly a first step but is most usefully considered as part of the initial-use stage. In addition many life-style users will eventually pass through a final stage characterized by re-entry into mainstream society either with, or without, abandoning the use of marijuana.

Initial use

Initial use refers to the first few, experimental, involvements with marijuana and is a relatively common phenomenon. Perhaps a majority of all college students in the USA and up to 40 per cent in Britain have tried marijuana as have significant minorities of non-college-educated youth (WHO, 1972; Young and Brooke-Crutchley, 1972; Plant, 1975). There are several factors that clearly predict initial use, many of which are the same factors which predict the initial use of drugs other than marijuana.

By far the strongest single predictor of whether or not a person will try marijuana is having friends who are users. Plant (1975) in a study

of 200 marijuana users in Cheltenham reported that over 90 per cent
of his sample had been introduced to the drug by friends or siblings
and only 5 per cent had first obtained it from strangers. Occasionally
a person may be induced to try marijuana as a result of direct social
pressure exerted by the peer group, but more often it occurs because
the person has observed that others he gets on with well have used
marijuana without deleterious consequences and is curious about the
effects it will have upon himself. So availability through friends and
the model of its use by friends are powerfully associated with a
person's own use of marijuana. One study of adolescents in New York
found that only 15 per cent of people did *not* try marijuana if their
best friends were users, whereas adolescents whose best friends did not
use marijuana were extremely unlikely to try it themselves (Kandel,
1973).

Just as involvement in what might be called a drug-using subculture
is predictive of marijuana use, so involvement in certain other subcultures is strongly predictive of non-use. This is particularly true of
involvement in organized religion. What is not clear is whether this
abstinence is because the same psychological needs which lead some
people to use drugs can be met by religious activity or whether strong
religious beliefs are effective inhibitors of illegal activities in general.
Indeed it may be that the conformity to traditional standards which is
often found in those people who practise religious observances in
Christian societies may be a sufficient explanation for their not
indulging in unconventional habits of any kind.

The same study (Kandel, 1973) highlighted another factor which is
associated with the likelihood of experimental marijuana use in young
people: the drug use patterns of their parents. While it is not the case
that the majority of marijuana users have parents who use, or have
used, marijuana there is evidence for what Goode (1975) has called
'generational continuity' in drug use. Parents who make regular use of
legal drugs like alcohol and tobacco are significantly more likely to
have children who use marijuana (as well as legal drugs) than are
parents who neither smoke nor drink. Indeed the extent of parental
use of patent medicines and drugs obtained on doctors' prescriptions
is correlated to some extent with the marijuana use of their offspring.
It is, perhaps, not unreasonable to suggest that parents provide a
model for their children which leads to a general pro-drug orientation. Their behaviour will appear to their children to be based upon
the belief that the use of chemicals to alter physical and psychological

states is a quite normal and acceptable part of life. It must appear as something of a contradiction to their children for the parents to condemn marijuana smoking while themselves happily using drugs such as alcohol which are, arguably, far more dangerous.

Other aspects of parental behaviour are also related to drug use in the next generation. As might be expected, family disorganization and instability, the absence of one or both parents, and over and under domination of children by parents are predictive of marijuana use in the offspring. What has also been revealed is that the style of family life even in stable and intact families influences the propensity of the offspring to use drugs. Families marked by a *laissez-faire* style of organization, families where the parents are relatively permissive and liberal in outlook, and families where short-range and self-indulgent goals are highly valued are more likely to find that their adolescent members try marijuana and other drugs (Gorsuch and Butler, 1976).

A reflection of similar characteristics has also been found in the personality of those who experiment with marijuana. They themselves are less conformist in outlook (or are sometimes said to have low super-ego strength), more likely to take left-wing views on political issues, and more likely to be cynical and disenchanted with the society in which they live. It has been pointed out, however, that as marijuana use becomes the norm rather than the exception in large segments of society the negative relationship between social conformity and use of the drug may disappear (Gorsuch and Butler, 1976).

Statistically marijuana users, like their parents, are much more likely to have used legal drugs, particularly alcohol and tobacco, than non-users. Even the use of coffee and aspirin is related in a crude statistical sense to the likelihood of a person's using marijuana (Goode, 1975, p. 434) as is having experienced a general anaesthetic (Blum *et al.*, 1970). Equally, it is true that people who experiment with marijuana are more likely to try other drugs such as heroin, amphetamines and LSD than are people without marijuana experience. This statistical relationship has led to the 'stepping-stone' fallacy achieving a certain currency. The theory that marijuana use leads to heroin use is clearly untenable. If the same argument were to be applied elsewhere in the drug 'chain', it could also be suggested that tobacco smoking causes marijuana use because virtually all marijuana users have previously smoked tobacco. Just as it is true that only a very small proportion of tobacco smokers become marijuana users, so only a small proportion of marijuana users become heroin addicts.

Research has shown that while practically all heroin addicts have used marijuana, only about 6 per cent of all marijuana users become heroin users (Gergen *et al.*, 1972 cited in Gorsuch and Butler, 1976).

There is much more reason to give credence to the hypothesis that a 'drug-prone' personality exists. The fact that a correlation exists between the likelihood of using any drug, legal or illegal, and the likelihood of using other drugs either serially or concurrently seems to suggest that certain people are much more prone to use drugs in general than are others. The evidence from Plant's (1975) study is very useful here. He actually concentrated on marijuana use but some idea of the range of drugs employed in his sample is given in Table 5.2. There is reason to think that the actual substance being used by those of a drug-taking disposition is more a matter of availability than anything else (Spear, 1969; Walker, 1972). Proneness to use drugs probably develops as a result of family experiences which produce a positive attitude to drugs combining with an above average need for stimulation and sensation seeking and a history of positive encounters with psychoactive chemicals.

Table 5.2   Multiple drug use by cannabis users

Percentage of cannabis users also using:	
Tobacco	81
Alcohol	90
LSD	77.5
Amphetamines	54
Barbiturates	30
Opium	32.5
Cocaine	13.5
Mescaline	26
Heroin	12
Other illegal drugs	11

Source: adapted from Plant (1975).

Combining several of the factors reviewed above, Johnson (1973) was able to achieve almost 100 per cent accuracy in predicting which individuals, among a large group of college students, would experiment with marijuana. The four factors he used as predicators were sex, religious orientation, political liberalism and tobacco smoking.

No fewer than 97 per cent of male, non-religious, liberal, cigarette smokers tried marijuana compared with less than 5 per cent of religious, conservative, women who did not smoke tobacco. The degree of accuracy in prediction is remarkable and clearly illustrates that 'the life style of certain segments of society *almost implies* marijuana use' (Goode, 1975, p. 421).

Regular use

For a large proportion, perhaps a majority, of people who experiment with marijuana, their involvement ends there. After a few encounters they either do not bother with the drug again or may indulge in occasional use at parties or other informal social gatherings. Other people, however, do go on to become more habitual users of marijuana and consequently have to invest some time and energy in securing supplies. The hurdles that have to be overcome in graduating from initial, experimental use to regular use were outlined in a seminal paper by Becker (1963). Firstly, the initiate must learn to smoke the marijuana cigarettes in the correct fashion to maximize the effect. This involves a somewhat different technique from tobacco smoking as more air must be taken in and the mixture must be held in the lungs for longer than would normally be done with tobacco smoke. Secondly, the user must learn to perceive the effects of the drug and link them with marijuana. We have already seen that the effects of marijuana are very subtle, to say the least, and the substance itself is frequently used in conjunction with alcohol and other drugs. In laboratory settings many people naïve to marijuana use have great difficulty in determining the effects of the drug or even recognizing that they have ingested it.

Thirdly, and most crucially, Becker points out that the incipient regular user must learn that the effects he has come to recognize, such as thirst, dizziness, confusion and fear, which objectively are ambiguous to say the least, are *subjectively* pleasurable. The common element in each of these three processes is, of course, learning. As already noted, smoking marijuana is universally a social activity and a typical pattern appears to be that more experienced users teach less experienced users to appreciate the drug, both indirectly by modelling but also directly and didactically by telling the novice how to smoke and what to expect.

The experimental users who fail to progress beyond this stage to become regular users are in a sense insufficiently socialized so to do. Orcutt (1975) has suggested that the perceived effects of marijuana are almost entirely symbolic: 'consensually defined conceptions of effects are learned and experienced by users as a function of social interaction with other users' (p. 1023). If the experimental user firmly believes that the effects of marijuana are being exaggerated by his peers and they are deluding themselves into believing that getting high is a real and pleasant experience then it is quite unlikely that he will get high. If, however, he comes to the situation with an appropriate set to become intoxicated and a willingness to accept the social influences of the more experienced users present then this makes subsequent use that much more likely.

There is experimental evidence for some of these propositions. Carlin *et al.* (1972) established two conditions under which marijuana was smoked by experienced users. In one condition the participants were told that a pill they had swallowed potentiated marijuana intoxication, and in the second condition that the pill attenuated intoxication, whereas, in fact, the pill was composed of an inert substance in both conditions. In addition an actor was introduced into the situation and instructed to simulate intoxication in condition one, and simulate sobriety in condition two. Estimates of the participants' degree of intoxication were obtained from several tests of cognitive and motor functioning and the results showed that, in the dosages in which it is normally used, the effects attributed to marijuana were heavily influenced by the set of the respondents and the social setting. Interestingly in a later study Carlin *et al.* (1974) found that people without experience of marijuana were much less likely to be influenced by people modelling intoxication than were the experienced users and were less well able to recognize their own intoxication. This was presumably both because the marijuana naïve students had self-selected to *not* use the drug previously and also because they had not passed through the previous socialization process and learned to label their feelings as intoxication.

Cappell and Pliner (1974) looked at the effect of cognitive variables on the amount of marijuana required to obtain intoxication in experimental conditions. They allowed the experienced users who formed their sample to smoke as much marijuana as they needed to achieve a 'nice high'. Each person was supplied with either large or small marijuana cigarettes which, unbeknown to them, varied in the concentration of THC they contained. The results showed that the participants were heavily influenced in their judgement of when they were satisfied by the number of 'joints' smoked irrespective of their size or potency. Thus at one extreme those people who were presented with large and potent cigarettes ingested three or four times more THC before they reported intoxication than those at the other extreme who were given the smaller, weaker cigarettes. This, perhaps more clearly than any other single study, shows the relative power of cognitive and experience variables compared to pharmacological variables in determining the subjective effects flowing from marijuana use.

Life-style use

The great majority of regular users either remain at this level of involvement or eventually scale down their use or even stop using marijuana altogether following distressing experiences produced by contaminated supplies or brushes with the law. The way in which a hard core of regular users can become so intensely involved with marijuana that it becomes the central feature of their lives has been explained most cogently by sociologists working within the labelling theory of deviance.

The labelling perspective starts by pointing out that deviance and social problems are created, not by a type of behaviour, but by society's reaction to that behaviour.

> Social groups create deviance by making rules whose infraction constitutes deviance, and by applying those rules to particular people and labeling them as outsiders. . . . The deviant is one to whom that label has successfully been applied; deviant behavior is behavior that people so label.   (Becker, 1963, p. 9)

The effects of successful public labelling are powerful both in terms of a changed reaction of others to the stigmatized deviant and, perhaps more importantly, of a change in the way the labelled person comes to perceive himself. This transformation may be superficial, temporary and specific, or it may produce a permanent and fundamental change in the person's whole self-identity and way of life.

Young (1971) provided a detailed analysis of the impact of being labelled as deviant in his study of the way in which society's stereotypes affected the social world of marijuana users in Notting Hill, London, in terms of what he calls 'deviancy amplification'. This process was mediated, in the case of these marijuana smokers, by the police as agents of the larger society. The following steps occurred in the process of deviancy amplification in his example:

(1) There exists a fairly clear-cut social stereotype of drug users. They are believed to be psychologically unstable, corrupted individuals without any sense of values, living a life of unbridled sexuality, enjoying only superficial relationships with others and whose whole existence is organized around drugs. In this stereotype, marijuana and the harder drugs are not distinguished. Incidentally, Young argues against the truth of this stereotype, but the accuracy of the picture it presents is largely irrelevant in assessing its impact on those affected by it.

(2) The police accept this stereotypic image and act towards users in accordance with it. The police are motivated to act against marijuana users because of public pressure and because of the moral indignation they feel towards those who flaunt the values which they themselves hold to most strongly − particularly masculinity, sobriety, respectability, conformity and a belief in the intrinsic value of work. In addition, of course, marijuana users are relatively soft targets for the police compared to some other, more traditional, types of criminal, and can sometimes be used to make police efficiency appear greater than it in fact is. From time to time therefore the police crack down on marijuana users.

(3) The drug-using group has to adapt to this situation, partly for self-protection, and partly as a response to a sense of injustice and of being misunderstood. The result is that the life-style of the marijuana users changes. They become more secretive, more segregated from wider society and will also begin to feel more affinity with other 'persecuted' groups such as hard drug users, blacks, homosexuals, criminals and so on. The social cohesiveness of the group will become strengthened and theories will evolve which explain why the group is being put under such pressure. These theories will inevitably be critical of the larger society, and will crystallize the independent value system of the members in opposition to that society. Continued police pressure may produce a scarcity of marijuana, or at least a rise in the price, and obtaining it will come to occupy a larger and larger share of each user's time and attention. In short, the original

stereotype gradually comes to be fulfilled. Fantasy is translated into reality, as Young puts it.

(4) As more aspects of the stereotype become fulfilled, and become visible − long hair, distinctive dress and alienation from ordinary work habits − a further response is evoked from the media, the public and, consequently, the police. It also becomes increasingly difficult for the deviant to abandon his way of life and return to straight society without giving up his whole, socially created, self-image.

(5) Having been confirmed in their stereotype of the drug user, the police may apply still more pressure. The drug users react again, and so a vicious circle is created. The initial, perhaps trivial, deviancy is amplified beyond all recognition. Increasingly both groups − society through the police and the marijuana users themselves − receive confirmation of their own perceptions of the situation. Eventually the two groups are so totally opposed that no *rapprochement* is possible, or even thought desirable, by either side.

In this way a genuine subculture develops in which marijuana is used more for its potency as a symbol of social opposition and group solidarity than for its real or imagined pharmacological properties. This distinguishes life-style users from the regular users who, while they may share some of the social definitions of the life-style users, basically use marijuana for recreational purposes and to get high, while maintaining an otherwise reasonably traditional way of life.

The question that remains is why should the larger society, through its agents the police, wish to persecute the marijuana smoker and label him as deviant? After all, it may be said, the only possible victims of their indulgence are the drug users themselves. A partial answer to this question may be found in the fact that one aspect of the stereotype that society has of drug users involves a virtual negation of culturally prescribed values. It is this which ensures a very strong reaction from conformists. Because marijuana users are thought to be threatening the basis of social convention and morality while at the same time actually enjoying themselves without having earned the right to do so, powerful resentment will be experienced by those who have accepted the social contract and traded their spontaneity for security. It is probably no coincidence that many key elements of the stereotype of drug users (idleness, self-indulgence, sexual licence and all forms of hedonism) are exactly the most repressed impulses in civilized society (Freud, 1961).

Heroin

It is common to contrast the British and American approach to dealing with the problem of heroin use (and indeed other narcotics). Since the 1914 Harrison Narcotics Act the use of heroin in the United States has been virtually outlawed. Because the possession and use of heroin is itself a criminal offence, most users have had to resort to raising the money they need to obtain illegal supplies of heroin by involvement in other kinds of criminal activity. In Britain, on the other hand, heroin addiction has been defined as a medical problem since the 1924 Rolleston Committee Report. From that time onward it has been possible for certain groups of physicians to supply heroin legally to people who are known to be addicted to the drug. Many authors (e.g. Brecher *et al.*, 1972; Schur, 1961) have suggested that the British approach has been far more successful in controlling the spread of heroin addiction than has the American approach. In terms of the figures relating to the number of addicts in the two countries, this conclusion is undoubtedly justified. Andima *et al.* (1973), extrapolating from the New York City Narcotics Register, estimated that in 1971 there were upwards of 426,000 heroin addicts in New York City alone. In the same year in Britain there were under 3000 people known to be addicted to all forms of narcotics (including methadone and cocaine).

Whatever the differences between these two approaches to the drug addiction problem, they are in fact based upon very similar assumptions about the origin of addiction. Both the criminal and medical models of how to respond to the question of addiction stem from a naïve belief in what has been called the 'bewitching power' of narcotics (Solomon and Marshall, 1973). The poverty of this approach to explaining narcotics addiction has only recently become apparent, although evidence of its inadequacy has been available for a long time. After a brief survey of the traditional approaches to explaining addiction, the remainder of this section will be devoted to developing a more satisfactory model of heroin addiction.

Traditional theories of addiction

An early and still current theory of heroin addiction is that of Lindesmith (1968) although the elements of this explanation are so simple as to hardly warrant the designation 'theory'. The potential addict is believed to pass through three stages in his relationship with the drug. At first the physical feelings associated with injection are mixed — some are pleasant, but many are unpleasant. Later research has shown that between 45 and 90 per cent of first-time users of heroin report basically unpleasant experiences. Even those destined to go on to become addicts are more likely to recount their first experience as being unpleasant, or a mixture of pleasant and unpleasant effects, than as being pleasant (McAuliffe, 1975). A number of people will discontinue their use of heroin after their first few encounters. Lindesmith suggests, however, that the unpleasant effects soon diminish and the experience of heroin use becomes totally pleasurable.

> Once you squeeze it in, the drug circulates with your blood, it will come round your system, and all of a sudden your eyes will feel like they gonna close up on you. You feel drowsy, your mouth will dry up on you, your spit will turn into cotton balls, right?; then you just start nodding all over the place, take out the works, clean 'em up, an' hide 'em. Then you got that boss feeling, man, like your own boss, there ain't nobody can tell you what to do in this world.
> (Hector Rodriguez, Drug addict, in Larner and Tefferteller, 1966)

The overwhelmingly pleasurable effects of heroin use mean that the potential addict begins to use the drug more frequently and more regularly. In a very short while (maybe only a week or two) Lindesmith suggests that physiological dependence develops. The most significant feature of dependence is that the incipient addict experiences very unpleasant physical symptoms when he is not using the drug. These are the well-known withdrawal symptoms associated with heroin (such things as extreme irritability, diarrhoea, anxiety, hypothermia, increased respiratory rate and depression). From this point on the use of heroin takes on a new meaning for the addict. It is no longer used to produce pleasant, euphoric effects but is used primarily to avoid the unpleasant effects of withdrawal. As Lindesmith says the desire for heroin is fixed by negative reinforcement. The unfortunate addict has been trapped by the initially overwhelmingly pleasant effects of heroin and now has to endure the agonies of withdrawal whenever supplies of the drug are unobtainable. It is purely to stave off these terrifying withdrawal effects that the addict keeps using the drug.

It is the central tenet of this theory then that the addict is not using heroin in order to achieve the euphoria that once accompanied its injection, although there is evidence that even chronic addicts do experience the euphoric effects of heroin (McAuliffe and Gordon, 1974).

A second type of theory of addiction which also relies on the pharmacological power of heroin as a central explanatory construct is the 'escape into oblivion' model. Under this general rubric are the explanations of addiction which suggest that the addict is motivated by a desire to escape from intolerable physical or social distress and seeks out heroin as a refuge. This type of explanation is obviously quite appropriate to the so-called medical addicts; patients who received morphine in a medical context to ease severe pain and who have become addicted subsequently. It may also be an appropriate genre of explanation for the medical practitioners and others associated with medicine, who may turn to opiates for relief from stress associated with overwork and so on. However the escape theory of addiction has received widespread currency in explaining the more common forms of addiction among people who are experiencing neither physical pain nor the stress of overwork − namely those who live in exceptionally deprived social circumstances.

Perhaps one of the earliest systematic attempts to use an escape model to explain addiction was that of Merton (1957). Merton bases his explanation of addiction (and a whole range of other deviant behaviours) on his concept of anomie. Anomie in Merton's terms arises from a disjunction between socially valued goals and socially approved means of achieving them. Thus in a society that inculcates a universally shared desire for material success, wealth and the good life, but which erects barriers that in practice prevent large segments of the population from achieving these cultural goals, the psychologically uncomfortable state of anomie will be created. Although Merton describes several ways in which individuals will attempt to cope with their anomic situation, the one that is relevant here is retreatism. Those who adapt by retreatism reject both the prevailing cultural goals and the socially approved means of achieving them: they are, sociologically speaking, true aliens. One response of the frustrated and handicapped individual who is doomed for ever to failure within society is to drop out and to attempt to escape from the requirements of that society. The most frequently used methods of escape according to Merton are psychosis, vagrancy, chronic alcoholism and drug addiction.

As with the sociological theory of addiction put forward by Linde-smith, the 'escape into oblivion' theories rely heavily on the powerful pharmacological properties of heroin in order to explain the hold that it can get over people. Fixing attention on the chemical itself rather than on the social meaning of drug use can be seen as the origin of both the British and the American approach to the prevention and treatment of addiction. Presumably because the authorities believe the drug to be far too powerful for most people to use sensibly, and because of its potential for producing extreme consequences for users, the American response has been to criminalize possession and use. The implicit hope is that this will limit the spread of use by making it difficult to obtain the drug and by imposing very severe sanctions on those who use it. The British approach, although it may be considered more humane in some ways, also accepts the assumption that heroin addicts are unfortunate victims of a very powerful substance. They are regarded as having an illness and therefore deserving the tra-ditional response given to people who are sick. This perspective has been reinforced by 'evidence' supporting the amazing addictive power of heroin and the vulnerability of the naïve to this power. We are all familiar with stories of pushers giving away free samples of heroin or lacing other drugs with it in order to secure the custom of future gen-erations of addicts. Equally current are tales of addicts so dependent on the drug that they deliberately attempt to induce non-users to become like themselves so that they can subsequently have a clientele to whom they can sell heroin in order to support their own expensive habit.

The remainder of this chapter will be devoted to exposing the in-adequacies of any biochemically based model of heroin addiction and offering an alternative understanding of drug use which relies on the social construction of the reality of the drug user and the psychologi-cal functions of being an 'addict'.

Inadequacy of biochemically based explanations

We have already seen that for many people their initial reaction to heroin is largely unpleasant; nevertheless, a proportion of people persist in using the drug even though they are by no means trapped into doing so on their first encounter. They must in some sense have been motivated to continue using the drug until they brought about their own entrapment. This as much as anything else exposes the naïvety of the trap and escape theories of addiction. One of the strongest stereotypes that pervades contemporary society from fictional accounts and from newspaper reports of actual occurrences is that of the strung-out, pathetic, degraded and unhappy drug addict. It cannot be the case that addiction arises from the improvidence of the unwary who fall under the influence of a drug of whose power they have no knowledge. In fact, of course, if we stand back for a moment from the actual problem of drug abuse we can agree with Blachly (1970) that humans have a particular predilection for self-destructive or, as he calls them, 'seductive' behaviours (for example smoking, suicide, delinquency, sex, gambling, alcoholism and rioting as well as drug abuse). Blachly suggests that these seductive behaviours have four prime qualities: the first of these is that the victim actively participates in his own victimization; secondly, the individual is fully aware of the potential adverse consequences of engaging in such behaviour; thirdly, the individual is also aware that there may be very considerable short-term gains from engaging in these behaviours; but fourthly, he or she is also aware that in the longer term these behaviours will produce negative consequences which far outweigh their short-term positive effects. Thus most excessive gamblers will readily agree that it is only the bookmakers who make money out of gambling; similarly most cigarette smokers are aware of the evidence that smoking is likely to shorten their life. Applying this analysis to heroin use, then, we may say that the potential addict is fully aware of the eventual consequences of his behaviour and is in a sense desirous of achieving these consequences.

Even without pointing to the obvious naïvety of the pharmacologically based explanations of addiction, sufficient evidence from other sources has gradually accumulated to indicate that any satisfactory model of addiction will have to take into account a range of known social factors which completely outweigh the importance of pharmacological aspects of the use of heroin. These additional factors will be reviewed in turn in order to be able to build on them subsequently when a social model of heroin addiction is developed.

The first fact to be considered here is one which has been known for a considerable period of time: that is, the very high relapse rate of addicts after apparently successful treatment. If pharmacological addiction is the basis of the problem rather than a symptom of something else, we would expect that when addicts are free of physiological dependence on heroin they should not necessarily have any more chance of becoming readdicted than anyone else. But this is clearly not the case. Siegel (1978) reports American studies which show that 90 per cent of all addicts entering treatment programmes relapse within one year; more importantly, 80 per cent of those who successfully complete the treatment programmes relapse very soon after discharge. These findings are by no means unique and reflect the common experience of those involved in drug programmes.

These data have to be articulated with what appears to be a completely contradictory set of findings which indicate that most addicts can spontaneously give up heroin. Robins (1980) noted that the use of heroin is rare in people aged over thirty and yet as most young addicts survive to this age they must at some point abandon their use of the drug. Robins cites a study done for the US National Institute on Drug Abuse which found that only 31 per cent of those men who had ever used heroin had done so in the last year. In other words, almost 70 per cent of one-time heroin users were currently not using the drug. Comparable figures for alcohol and tobacco showed that virtually all one-time users were current users and for other illegal drugs, such as marijuana, the majority of users continued using the drug. In fact there was much more movement out of heroin use than for any other single drug examined. But this movement away from heroin was certainly not because of therapeutic intervention. Several researchers have observed that even long-term addicts eventually reach a stage when they are able to give up their use of heroin with relatively little trouble. For example Frykholm (1979) found that the main reason given by ex-addicts for abandoning heroin was 'they were tired of the life of a street addict'. None of the 58 ex-addicts interviewed gave treatment or any form of therapy as their reason for abandoning heroin. In fact one of the best ways of achieving a stable, drug-free life following addiction appears to be to gain employment as a therapist in a drug treatment programme. This seems to indicate that a successful way of achieving abstinence from heroin is to substitute for the life-style of the addict an equally satisfying social role.

Further support for this idea has come from a number of studies of the experience of US soldiers in Vietnam and their subsequent history upon their return to the United States. Many servicemen had easy access to cheap, local supplies of heroin and took advantage of the opportunity to escape the boredom and horror around them. This not unnaturally led to considerable fears on the part of the military authorities that upon their return to the United States a flood of addicts would be discharged into the civilian population. Robins (1980) studied 1000 US servicemen returning from Vietnam and found that 50 per cent had used heroin while abroad and 25 per cent had used it regularly. Given the relative purity of the heroin they were using and the regularity of use, there is little doubt that many of these soldiers would have become physically dependent on heroin. Three years after their return to the United States only 2 per cent of the cohort were still using narcotics. This figure was very similar to the proportion of a matched sample of male non-veterans who had never left the United States. What this shows is that virtually all of the people who had been regular users of heroin were able to abandon it once their social situation became normalized. Physical dependence was no real obstacle to giving up heroin once the psychological need for it had been removed.

Account must also be taken of the reaction of foreign addicts who, from time to time, have come to Britain to take advantage of what they believe to be the virtually free supplies of pure heroin available by those who simply register as addicts with the National Health Service. In the early 1960s a significant proportion of new addicts known about officially in Britain were in fact from Canada, the United States and other foreign countries and they were being pre-scribed free heroin (Brecher *et al.*, 1972, p. 124). However it appears that many did not remain in Britain for very long.

A follow-up study of ninety-one Canadian addicts in Britain found that most of them had returned to Canada within a few years (Solomon, 1977, p. 16). The reason that the majority of them had done so was that they found they were missing the 'street life' — the hustling, contacts, making connections and so on. Here was a group who had firmly believed that heroin was the most important thing in their lives but who quickly discovered that the psychological significance of being an addict went far beyond having ready access to heroin. Indeed in some ways having access was just what they did not want as it removed the necessity for the clandestine life-style which had previously seemed to be an unfortunate, but inevitable, accompaniment of addiction but which emerged as the *raison d'être* of many addicts.

The same factors are probably operating in the changed pattern of heroin addiction among native British addicts. It is assumed that for many potential addicts the initial source of their supplies was other addicts who had excess legally obtained heroin to sell or share. Following the tightening up of prescription procedures in 1968, an alternative black market supplying 'Chinese' heroin from Hong Kong emerged and has become well established (Geraghty, 1972). At first glance it is not easy to understand how this market is maintained; the heroin it supplies is very expensive, undoubtedly impure, and its clients are eligible for free, pure heroin, or a substitute, if they register with a doctor at an NHS drug clinic. Many addicts appear to prefer to obtain their supplies illegally with all the attendant difficulties and dangers this involves. Again it is difficult to avoid the conclusion that the drug itself is peripheral to the whole enterprise of being an addict.

Finally we can turn to the most compelling evidence of all that heroin addiction means much more than the regular use of heroin. Perhaps somewhat belatedly, researchers have begun to look at exactly what substances 'heroin' addicts use when they obtain their illegal supplies. Primm and Bath (1973), for example, calculated the actual composition of heroin sold on the streets in New York City from data collected both by themselves and by earlier researchers. It appears that while the *mean* amount of heroin in samples bought on the street is between 10 per cent and 20 per cent, the *modal* or typical proportion is only about 0.5 per cent. More than half of all the street samples that were tested contained even less than 0.5 per cent of heroin with a large percentage containing none at all. Those who sell heroin on the illegal market make the maximum profit by selling bags of 'heroin' which usually contain little or no heroin but which occasionally, and unpredictably, contain a relatively high proportion. This intermittent supply of larger doses of real heroin may account for a proportion of deaths from overdoses: addicts may be convinced that their tolerance is greater than it in fact is because they have been using large quantities of other substances in the belief that they are heroin. A review of a large number of street drug analysis programmes in the US (Brown and Malone, 1974) confirmed findings that most 'heroin' sold on the black market is something else (whereas virtually all marijuana sold is what it claims to be) and strongly supports Primm and Bath's view that true heroin addiction in the physiological sense is perhaps rarer than previously believed and that 'pseudoheroinism' is a more accurate term to describe this habit pattern.

The other, equally fascinating, aspect of Primm and Bath's results concerned the actual constituents of street heroin. The contaminants of street heroin are by no means inert, cheap materials like talcum powder, as is often supposed. The most common contaminant found was quinine, which was in fact more common than pure heroin itself. The addition of quinine to heroin for injection was originally believed to be a precaution against the spread of malaria by unsterile syringes but it has now become the standard and relatively cheap way of diluting heroin. Other contaminants found in samples of street heroin include sodium bicarbonate, cocaine, nicotine, cyanide and sulphuric acid. Now the important point here is that many of the aspects of addiction that have been assumed to be caused by heroin are more likely to be secondary to quinine toxicity or to be related to some of the rarer contaminants of street heroin. It may be, for example, that it is quinine which produces the characteristic 'tracks' on the skin at the site of injection.

The use of non-inert contaminants must be primarily to convince the customer that he/she is actually buying heroin. Certainly some of the substances used to cut or entirely replace heroin will produce detectable physiological responses following injection. However heroin addicts also anticipate that there will be unpleasant side-effects such as abscesses and vein tracks and the smart pusher caters for these expectations too.

Again it is necessary to draw a distinction between the situation which prevails in the United States and the situation in Britain where many addicts receive pure heroin under medical supervision. As already pointed out, however, there may be a tendency for addicts and potential addicts to reject legal supplies in favour of illegal and inevitably contaminated supplies. In any case, the British practice of maintaining addicts on heroin or methadone may produce longer-term and genuine physical addiction and make it more difficult for the British addict to terminate a drug career than is the case in the United States (Wille, 1981).

All the factors reviewed in this section lead inexorably to the conclusion that the importance of heroin as a drug of abuse lies more in its social and symbolic meaning than in its pharmacological properties. The question becomes: to what are heroin addicts addicted if it is not heroin?

A social psychological explanation of heroin use: the role of addict

Several authors, in attempting to account for the inadequacy of traditional models of addiction, have used ideas such as those of a positive and often conscious motivation to become an addict (Jacobs, 1976).

It is this positive motivation which enables potential addicts to persist when faced by the unpleasant effects of initial heroin use, to relapse after detoxification, to suffer the negative personal, legal and social consequences of their behaviour, and to continue with their addiction even in the absence of their chosen drug. Equally, stopping heroin use is much more likely to follow the loss of this motivation, or the substitution of an alternative motivation, than it is to follow medical or psychiatric intervention.

It has become clear that what many addicts are seeking is not the euphoria of heroin intoxication (although they may believe this to be the case) but the socially validated identity of drug addict. This implies that there exists a well-defined and well-recognized social role of addict and that certain people at certain times in their lives find this role preferable to other, alternative roles. A role is defined in social psychology as a 'set of required or expected behaviors of people occupying a certain position in a group' (Stang, 1981, p. 98) and a good case can be made that 'drug addict' meets this definition quite well. The role of addict can be learned in just the same way as any other role and to the extent that it is providing reinforcements and satisfactions for those playing the role, it will persist.

Chein was one of the first authors to describe systematically the positive psychological functions that being a heroin addict served for the occupant of the role. He developed an explanation in terms of a contrast between the levels of status, control, feelings of mastery and competence which potential addicts experienced prior to their addiction with those achieved afterwards. According to Chein, the addict has usually failed to achieve a psychologically satisfactory social identity in straight society because he has from childhood been led to believe in his own incompetence. Hence he has been unable to find a vocation or any other 'meaningful, sustained activity around which he could, so to say, wrap his life' (1969, p. 23). Addiction offers a solution, not in terms of an escape into oblivion, but by providing a socially validated role that allows for the possibility of success and status within its own definitions.

The role of an addict is in many ways like any other job or vocation and carries many of the same responsibilities, obligations, and rewards. Jahoda and Rush (1980) have suggested that ordinary paid employment inevitably produces five latent functions: 1. Work imposes a structure on the working day. 2. Work compels people to come into contact with others. 3. Work demonstrates that some goals require collective action. 4. Work compels people to be more or less active. 5. Work confers a social identity (e.g. teacher, carpenter). The occupation of 'addict' (that is street addict) can quite clearly serve these same functions. The addict must organize his daily life so that supplies of heroin can be obtained and this is invariably through contacts with others in the drug scene. Obtaining supplies requires complex and co-operative collective action especially if the danger of arrest is to be minimized. Hustling to obtain money and maintain connections certainly requires the addict to have periods of almost frantic activity. But it is the final latent function of being an addict which is most important — that of offering a distinctive identity with well-defined role requirements, expectations and meanings.

Not only does the addict achieve a well-recognized identity in his own eyes and those of others but he also has the opportunity to achieve status. He almost invariably gets involved with an addict subculture in which he is accepted and can feel at home as he learns how to behave. His standing within this community is enhanced as he becomes more experienced, learns the appropriate language and customs, and begins to acquire the distinctive characteristics of an experienced junkie (Winick, 1974, p. 113). These include: needle marks along veins on the upper forearm; demonstrated skill in hustling money and making connections with heroin suppliers; experience of managing overdoses in other addicts; possession of a 'set of works' (spoon, heat source, syringe, etc.); a record of trouble with the police perhaps including some time spent in prison; and finally, reported experience of withdrawal symptoms if heroin is unavailable (Nurco *et al.*, 1981; Sackman *et al.*, 1978). Thus the addict's status is enhanced by the social visibility of his success in playing the role of addict in a professional and competent fashion. The actual use of heroin will occupy only a very minor part of his time, far more of which will be spent in obtaining supplies, evading the law and in encounters with other addicts. Talking about these daily experiences will also be rewarded by the respect and admiration of others within the subculture.

Kaplan has examined some of the psychological aspects of the reasons for choosing addiction as a way of life (Kaplan, 1972; Kaplan and Meyerowitz, 1970). He suggests that one of the most powerful motives in the human adult is the need to develop and maintain positive self-esteem and to avoid self-devaluing attitudes and that the adoption of a career as an addict is directly related to satisfying this need. Beginning with the observation that in the United States addicts are most likely to be found in areas characterized by low income, poor education, overcrowding, broken homes, and a high proportion of ethnic minorities, Kaplan suggests that the potential addict experiences a range of factors which are destructive of self-esteem from the earliest times in his life. The attitudes of others towards the individual to a large extent condition his attitude towards himself, so if others are perceived as having a poor opinion of the person this will lower his own self-esteem. In addition self-derogation will occur when the individual lacks qualities which he believes to be important, or fails to achieve the standards and goals which he sets for himself. Kaplan proposes that those people who have developed negative self-attitudes will be likely to adopt a deviant life-style of one form or another, particularly if the normative environment is associated with their self-devaluation and the available deviant patterns appear to have a high subjective probability of resulting in positive self-attitudes (Kaplan, 1972, p. 596). Should one of the alternatives available to the person be the addict subculture, and should this subculture enable the person to promote a positive self-attitude, then he will tend to become integrated into this form of adjustment. We have already seen how status in the eyes of others, and hence the possibility at least of self-esteem, may be gained within a drug subculture through routes which sharply diverge from, but are analogous to, those used in achieving status in the dominant, legitimate culture. Some people will try the heroin addict role and find that this too is an unsuitable method of achieving what they want and they will move on to yet other alternatives such as crime, alcohol, dropping out, even suicide perhaps (Kaplan, 1972). Sufficient people will, however, find the rewards of addiction psychologically satisfying to maintain a distinctive and viable alternative subculture.

The explanation of heroin addiction in terms of a social role adopted for the purpose of enhancing self-esteem seems to be much more compatible with the evidence relating to the natural history of drug abuse than do any of the pharmacologically based explanations. Because addicts are in fact often using heroin in a symbolic fashion, they are content with adulterated supplies so long as these are obtained in the time-honoured fashion. The Canadian heroin addicts who tried life in Britain lost the meaning of life as an addict when obtaining supplies became a routine, bureaucratic experience. Some British addicts too have preferred to avoid the tedious but secure round of doctors' waiting rooms, medical checks and queuing in high street chemist shops and have sought instead the excitement of obtaining illegal supplies, however insecure and squalid this may be. The US soldiers in Vietnam provide an example of a group of people who were actually using heroin for its pharmacological effects rather than because they were motivated to become addicts and they apparently found little difficulty in abandoning it when the need for a chemically induced escape disappeared. The person who is addicted to being an addict, on the other hand, finds it impossible to give up heroin use until something equally satisfying is available. This alternative may arise spontaneously, for example through marriage, children or perhaps a job (Ramos and Gould, 1978), or may occasionally be produced in a therapeutic context. Treatment programmes which place heavy emphasis on the power of heroin (such as methadone maintenance and detoxification schemes) are likely to fail. If addiction is regarded as an occupation, coming off heroin is equivalent to losing a job and the obvious solution is to find alternative employment. This is perhaps why treatment provided by therapeutic communities (such as Synanon House and its derivatives) are more successful (Van Ryswk *et al.*, 1981). After physical withdrawal the patients are immersed in a community of ex-addicts often without professional help. Life in the community is a round of work, education and many group sessions akin to encounter groups which provide a basis for the members to define and develop alternative social identities. The therapeutic community appears to work well because it leads to involvement, a new role and a new status which enable the ex-addict to develop new social skills and a new self-confidence without drugs. There is also an informal but powerful form of social control which reduces the likelihood of resumption of drug use because most of those involved come to value membership highly and therefore are prepared to adhere to the rules of the community. Although it has been suggested that this is substituting one form of addiction for another and many successful patients do go on to become involved in drug treatment and prevention programmes so do not completely abandon the drug scene, many other members are able to use therapeutic communities as a basis for creating a satisfactory drug-free personal identity.

References

Andima, H., Krug, D., Bergner, L., Patrick, S. and Whitman, S. (1973) A prevalence estimation model of narcotics addiction in New York City. *American Journal of Epidemiology* 98: 56−62.

Becker, H. S. (1963) *Outsiders: Studies in the Sociology of Deviance*. New York: The Free Press.

Blachly, P. H. (1970) *Seduction: A Conceptual Model in the Drug Dependencies and Other Contagious Ills*. Springfield, Ill.: Charles C. Thomas.

Blum, R. and Associates (1970) *Students and Drugs*. San Francisco: Jossey-Bass.

Brecher, E. M. and Editors of Consumers' Reports (1972) *Licit and Illicit Drugs*. New York: Consumers' Union.

Brown, J. K. and Malone, M. H. (1974) A street drug analysis program – three years later. In J. A. Marshman (ed.) *Street Drug Analysis*. Toronto: Alcoholism and Drug Addiction Research Foundation.

Cappell, H. and Pliner, P. (1974) Regulation of the self-administration of marihuana by psychological and pharmacological variables. *Psychopharmacologia 40*: 65–76.

Carlin, A. S., Bakker, C. B., Halpern, L. and Post, R. D. (1972) Social facilitation of marijuana intoxication: impact of social set and pharmacological activity. *Journal of Abnormal Psychology 80*: 132–40.

Carlin, A. S., Post, R. D., Bakker, C. B. and Halpern, L. M. (1974) The role of modeling and previous experience in the facilitation of marijuana intoxication. *Journal of Nervous and Mental Disease 159*: 275–81.

Chein, I. (1969) Psychological functions of drug abuse. In H. Steinberg (ed.) *Scientific Basis of Drug Dependence*. London: J. & A. Churchill.

Cohen, S. (1972) *Folk Devils and Moral Panics*. London: McGibbon & Kee.

Cooperstock, R. and Lennard, H. L. (1979) Some social meanings of tranquilizer use. *Sociology of Health and Illness 1*: 331–47.

Freud, S. (1961) *Civilization and Its Discontents*. Translated by J. Strachey. New York: W. W. Norton Inc.

Frykholm, B. (1979) Termination of the drug career. *Acta Psychiatrica Scandinavica 59*: 370–80.

Galanter, M., Stillman, R., Wyatt, J., Vaughan, T. B., Weingartner, H. and Nurnberg, F. L. (1974) Marihuana and social behaviour. *Archives of General Psychiatry 30*: 518–21.

Geraghty, T. (1972) Has 'Chinese' heroin put up the addict figures? *Sunday Times*, 19 March, p. 4.

Gergen, M. K., Gergen, K. J. and Morse, S. J. (1972) Correlates of marijuana use among college students. *Journal of Applied Social Psychology 2*: 1–16.

Goode, E. (1975) Sociological aspects of marijuana use. *Contemporary Drug Problems*, Winter, 397–445.

Gorsuch, R. L. and Butler, M. C. (1976) Initial drug abuse: a review of predisposing social psychological factors. *Psychological Bulletin 83*: 120–37.

Harré, R. (1979) *Social Being*. Oxford: Blackwell.

Hollister, L. E. (1971) Current research on marijuana. *Journal of Social Issues* 27: 23–34.

Irwin, S. (1973) A rational approach to drug abuse prevention. *Contemporary Drug Problems 2*: 3–46.

Jacobs, P. E. (1976) Epidemiology abuse: epidemiological and psychological models of drug abuse. *Journal of Drug Issues 6*: 113–22.

Jahoda, M. and Rush, H. (1980) *Work, Employment and Unemployment: An Overview of Ideas and Research Results in the Social Science Literature.* Science Policy Research Unit, Occasional Paper Series no. 12.

James, I. P. (1967) Suicide and mortality amongst heroin addicts in Britain. *British Journal of Addictions 62*: 391–8.

Johnson, B. D. (1973) *Marihuana Users and Drug Subcultures.* New York: John Wiley & Sons.

Kandel, D. (1973) Adolescent marijuana use: role of parents and peers. *Science 181*: 1067–70.

Kaplan, H. B. (1972) Toward a general theory of psychosocial deviancy: the case of aggressive behaviour. *Social Science and Medicine 6*: 593–617.

Kaplan, H. B. and Meyerowitz, J. H. (1970) Social and psychological correlates of drug abuse. *Social Science and Medicine 4*: 203–25.

Koumjian, K. (1981) The use of valium as a form of social control. *Social Science and Medicine 15E*: 245–9.

Larner, J. and Tefferteller, R. (1966) *The Addict in the Street.* London: Penguin Books.

Lindesmith, A. R. (1968) *Addiction and Opiates* (2nd edn). Chicago: Aldine Press.

McAuliffe, W. E. (1975) A second look at first effects: the subjective effects of opiates on non-addicts. *Journal of Drug Issues 5*: 369–99.

McAuliffe, W. E. and Gordon, R. A. (1974) A test of Lindesmith's theory of addiction: the frequency of euphoria among long-term addicts. *American Journal of Sociology 79*: 795–840.

Merton, R. K. (1957) *Social Theory and Social Structure.* Glencoe, Ill.: The Free Press.

Nurco, D. N., Cisin, I. H. and Balter, M. B. (1981) Addict careers. III. Trends across time. *The International Journal of the Addictions 16*: 1357–72.

Orcutt, J. D. (1975) Social determinant of alcohol and marijuana effects: a systematic theory. *International Journal of the Addictions 10*: 1021–33.

Plant, M. A. (1975) *Drugtakers in an English Town.* London: Tavistock Publications.

Primm, B. J. and Bath, P. E. (1973) Pseudoheroinism. *International Journal of the Addictions 8*: 231–42.

Ramos, M. and Gould, L. C. (1978) Where have all the flower children gone? A 5 year follow-up of a natural group of drug users. *Journal of Drug Issues 8*: 75–84.

Robins, L. N. (1980) The natural history of drug abuse. *Acta Psychiatrica Scandinavica*, Supplement 284, *62*: 7–20.

Royal College of Psychiatrists (1979) *Alcohol and Alcoholism*. London: Tavistock Publications.

Sackman, B. S., Sackman, M. M. and Deangelis, G. G. (1978) Heroin addiction as an occupation. *International Journal of the Addictions 13*: 427–42.

Schur, E. M. (1961) British narcotics policies. *Journal of Criminal Law, Criminology and Police Science 51*: 619–29.

Siegel, S. (1978) The role of conditioning in drug tolerance and addiction. In J. D. Keehn (ed.) *Psychopathology in Animals*. New York: Academic Press.

Solomon, E. and Marshall, W. L. (1973) A comprehensive model for the acquisition, maintenance and treatment of drug taking behaviour. *British Journal of Addiction 68*: 215–20.

Solomon, R. (1977) The evolution of non-medical opiate use in Canada. *Drug Forum – The Journal of Human Issues 6*: 1–26.

Spear, H. B. (1969) The growth of heroin addiction in the United Kingdom. *British Journal of Addiction 64*: 245–55.

Stang, D. J. (1981) *Introduction to Social Psychology*. Belmont, Calif. Brooks/Cole.

Stark, R. (1975) *Social Problems*. New York: Random House.

Stefanis, C., Dornbush, R. and Fink, M. (eds) (1977) *Hashish: Studies of Long-term Use*. New York: Raven Press.

Van Ryswk, C., Churchill, M., Velasquez, J. and McGuire, R. (1981) Effectiveness of halfway home placement for alcohol and drug abusers. *American Journal of Drug and Alcohol Abuse 8*: 499–512.

Verbrugge, L. M. (1982) Sex differences in legal drug use. *Journal of Social Issues 38*: 59–76.

Walker, M. (1972) Research blow at 'drugs ladder' theory. *Guardian*, 10 October, p. 12.

Weil, A. T., Zinberg, N. E. and Nelson, J. M. (1968) Clinical and psychological effects of marijuana in man. *Science 162*: 1234–42.

Wille, R. (1981) Ten-year follow-up of a representative sample of London heroin addicts: clinic attendance, abstinence and mortality. *British Journal of Addiction 76*: 259–66.

Winick, C. (1974) Some aspects of careers of chronic heroin users. In E. Josephson and E. E. Carroll (eds) *Drug Use: Epidemiological and Sociological Approaches*. New York: John Wiley and Sons.

World Health Organization (1972) The use of cannabis. *World Health Organization Chronicle 26*: 20–8.

Young, J. (1971) The role of the police as amplifiers of deviancy, negotiators of reality and translators of fantasy: some consequences of our present system of drug control as seen in Notting Hill. In S. Cohen (ed.) *Images of Deviance*. London: Penguin Books.

Young, J. and Brooke-Crutchley, J. (1972) Student drug use. *Drugs and Society 1*: 11–15.

Zacune, J. and Hensman, C. (1971) *Drugs, Alcohol and Tobacco in Britain*. London: Heinemann.

6 Drugs and human memory

C. M. Smith

Theoretical and methodological issues

Introduction

It has been known for a long time that drugs can affect memory. Probably drugs affecting the cholinergic system have the longest association with effects on memory and are still the major focus of interest. It became recognized early that some varieties of solanaceous plants containing the anticholinergic drugs atropine and scopolamine caused bizarre mental states, when eaten. The ancient Greeks used a variety of the plant hyoscyamus to evoke prophecies. In the seventeenth century there are anecdotal reports of the effects of these drugs on memory. In 1676 an incident of mass poisoning with datura stramonium occurred in Virginia. Some British troops cooked the plant as a food, and for up to several days displayed strange behaviour and had amnesia for the whole episode. At the beginning of this century scopolamine was first used in obstetrics in combination with morphine by Gauss and produced *Dämmerschlaf* or 'twilight sleep'. This was recognized as a state in which the patient was able to respond appropriately to stimuli which were not remembered later. In subsequent clinical practice scopolamine was used for premedication before surgical anaesthesia. It soon became widely recognized that there was an increased incidence of amnesia for events preceding the operation in patients treated with the drug.

Many studies have been carried out in the last twenty years to investigate this effect of anticholinergic and other drugs on memory. During this time drug studies have become less empirical and more based on a theoretical framework. This framework has evolved from studies on both animals and man. Drugs in turn have proved useful tools to contribute to knowledge about both the psychological structure and biochemical substrates of memory. Recently this approach, together with knowledge of neuropsychological deficits and biochemical lesions in various memory disorders, has prompted rational attempts to improve disordered memory, using drugs. For clarity, the following account is divided into experimental and clinical sections. However, the reader will realize that there are strong links between them.

Theories of human memory

One of the most useful ways of conceptualizing the memory system has been the information processing model originally proposed by Broadbent in 1958 in his theories about attention. This model has since been developed by many workers and has been described as the 'modal model' because of its general acceptance among psychologists. The most popular elaboration of this model has been produced by Atkinson and Shiffrin (1971).

Information first enters a series of registers each limited to a single modality, and is then passed first to a short-term store, and then after further processing to long-term storage. The system structure consists of these three memory stores and the passive transfer of information between them. Information decays fairly quickly in the sensory and short-term store and much more slowly in the long-term store. The short-term store is the centre of a control system which uses various control processes to direct the flow of information in the memory system. These control processes include coding procedures and rehearsal and retrieval strategies. Coding is seen as an important control process whereby relevant associations from long-term storage are activated and registered in the short-term store together with incoming information.

The design and interpretation of most drug studies have been based on this type of model. Attention has been focused firstly on a primary or short-term memory structure which retains small amounts of information for brief periods of time and secondly on long-term memory which involves the acquisition of larger amounts of information and retention for longer periods of time. Thirdly the effects of drugs on retrieval processes involved in recovery of information from long-term storage has received some attention. Generally less interest has been shown in the interaction of drugs with the active control processes elaborated by Atkinson and Shiffrin. However, effects of drugs on coding of information has been explored in some recent studies. There is usually a time-lag between development of pure theory and its practical application in other areas. Some more recent theoretical developments, for example Baddeley and Hitch's (1974) elaboration of short-term memory, or 'working memory', have not been explored and the effects of drugs on memory have therefore not yet been studied in the context of cognition in general. Likewise the concept of semantic memory has not captured the imagination of psychopharmacologists. It was Tulving (1972) who made the important distinction between semantic and episodic memory. He defined semantic memory as 'a system for receiving, retaining and transmitting information about meaning of words, concepts and classification of concepts' and episodic memory as 'memory for personal experiences and their temporal relations'. Drug studies still exist mainly in the realm of traditional memory represented by episodic memory and free-recall paradigms. This may change but at the moment the interest usually revolves round how a drug affects recall or recognition of a small piece of information supplied by the experimenter.

Experimental drug studies

Techniques used to assess the effects of drugs on memory have been diverse. In some early clinically based studies of anticholinergic drugs, memory for incidental natural events was usually assessed, e.g. memory for procedures in the operating theatre. There was no attempt at standardization of the stimulus or checking that subjects had paid attention to it. Not surprisingly, although amnesic effects were demonstrated these were often modest and their magnitude varied from study to study. When systematic experimental studies were conducted within a more theoretical framework, paradigms from experimental psychological studies were adopted, for example: free recall of word lists, serial learning, paired-associate learning and recognition of words, designs and pictures.

Depending on the design of the drug study, alternate forms of memory tests are usually required. The above tasks have the advantages that they are easily scored and equivalent alternate forms can usually be generated, provided that care is taken in the case of word lists to match forms of the test appropriately for properties including concreteness, frequency, and association value. It is more difficult to arrange equivalent forms of non-verbal material. In any event, particularly with more complex material, it is desirable to carry out pilot studies to check equivalence of forms of the test. The above techniques only involve the presentation of separate items. Alternate forms of tests to investigate the effects of drugs on memory for short sentences, prose and composite pictures require a great deal of care to achieve standardization and develop reliable scoring methods. For this reason, some psychometric tests, for example the Wechsler memory scale, have proved a useful source of test material, provided that their limitations in standardization and scoring techniques are appreciated. In general, however, psychometric tests are not a good source of test material as some of the tests employ rather idiosyncratic material. Some paradigms recently developed for use in neuropsychological studies are more useful. Buschke (1973) used a selective reminding procedure which involved learning a list of words over several trials, with subjects being prompted only with words which they had failed to recall on the previous trial. This ingenious technique appears to allow some separation of drug effects on storage and retrieval.

The number of alternate forms of tests required can be minimized by the use of an independent group design rather than a crossover study. For this reason independent group designs are frequently used. However large between-subject variance in memory ability can then pose problems. Following matching for age, pilot studies to screen for proficiency in memory tasks are desirable, as subject characteristics which predict memory ability have been little investigated. In one study with medical students we incidentally discovered that students with high marks in anatomy examinations perform rather well on free recall of word lists!

The careful choice and interpretation of tests and also the selection of methods of retention tests, e.g. by free recall, cued recall or recognition, allow insight into the nature of the effect of a drug on memory. Also the time at which the drug is administered in relation to presentation of material and retention testing can provide information about the mechanism of action of the drug. If a drug is administered before the learning trial, any change in subsequent retention should be cautiously interpreted as the drug may have an influence on a number of processes, apart from memory, including perception, attention and motivation. This can be investigated to some extent by a battery of psychological tasks including memory and non-memory tests, in an attempt to localize the drug effect to memory processes. If a drug is administered after the learning trial, then any effect on retention is traditionally ascribed to an effect on memory processes. In animal studies, drugs have been administered at various times after learning in order to examine the effects of drugs on consolidation of the memory trace, but this variable has received little attention in human studies where drug administration has usually closely and conveniently followed presentation of material.

Drugs have been administered by a variety of routes, orally, intravenously, intramuscularly and subcutaneously. The oral route is the most convenient but suffers from the drawback of a lag in onset of drug effect which can be very variable, depending on several factors including the presence of food in the stomach and intestine. For an early, consistent response, the intravenous route is the best choice but this can be dangerous with some drugs. The intramuscular or subcutaneous route is therefore often chosen. These are usually safer than the intravenous route and the response is reasonably consistent. More recently one or two studies have employed 'slow intravenous infusions'. This approach, when feasible, is to be encouraged as it can allow for steady-state drug levels to be obtained. It is often desirable to present tasks in a fixed order, for example when testing retention of the same material by recall and recognition. In this situation, if a single dose of drug was administered in a traditional way with a rising and falling concentration phase, differential drug effects could easily reflect the availability of the drug rather than a selective drug effect on recognition or recall. Chronic drug dosing can also be used to achieve sustained plasma levels of drug. However, few such studies have yet been carried out. It is rational for single dose studies to be made in the first instance, as tolerance may occur to the effects of a drug after chronic dosing. In experimental studies this would mean information would be lost about the potential of the drug to affect memory mechanisms. However, in clinical studies it is of practical importance to establish early any waning of drug effect after chronic treatment as this would be a limiting factor in developing the drug as a therapeutic agent.

Clinical drug studies

In evaluating the effects of drugs on patients with memory disorder, many of the above points on measures and design are applicable. Indeed it can be argued strongly that initial studies on patients should be conducted in the laboratory setting using structured memory tests. Further, it is only when such studies look promising that a clinical trial of the drug should be launched to investigate therapeutic effects. This is because in assessing effects on behaviour in everyday life the use of rating scales and similar tools is very difficult. Many variables which are difficult to control loom large and any beneficial or other effects are difficult to observe. Even in the laboratory setting, studies with patients present many problems. Within-patient studies are usually preferable as severity of memory disorder and other additional cognitive problems are very variable. However, in degenerative disorders like Alzheimer's disease, evaluating treatments against a changing baseline can complicate matters.

Choice of memory test is another important issue. It is not worthwhile assessing the effects of a drug on an aspect of memory when we know from experimental studies that the drug is unlikely to affect it. More importantly it is not fruitful to investigate drug effects on areas of patient's memory functioning which appear intact. This appears fairly obvious but is often overlooked.

The whole question of the validity of measures used needs very careful consideration. Word lists may prove useful as these are relatively easy to prepare and score. However attempts should be made to present meaningful material. Word lists might take the form of a shopping list or checklist of items to pack for a holiday. Also memory for connected prose material merits inclusion in the test battery, provided it has face validity and appears as if it might be of some interest to the patient. At the moment common sense in choosing tests is the best guide. However, preliminary studies suggest that memory for prose passages may show the best correlation with everyday memory difficulties. This is not the place to discuss the myriad problems of clinical trials in memory disorder. Several have been attempted and some of the required methodology is being sorted out. A lot of further effort will be necessary in developing rating scales which evaluate symptoms of memory deficit, which are specifically related to the various syndromes of memory disorder. Also, it is increasingly being realized that it may be necessary to administer treatments alongside retraining or other forms of non-drug therapy. This is not a revolutionary idea. Even with the often effective drug l-dopa, some exercise is required before the patient with Parkinson's disease can make full use of his improvement in mobility.

Experimental investigations

Drugs affecting cholinergic synapses

Anticholinergic drugs   Anticholinergic drugs have been studied more extensively than other types of drug for their effects on memory. Following the observation that scopolamine appeared to cause amnesia when given pre-operatively, several experimental studies were carried out in the clinical setting. Hardy and Wakely (1962) found some amnesia for a standard visual stimulus and events following scopolamine treatment, but little effect with atropine, when these drugs were given in normal clinical dosage, combined with morphine. Pandit and Dundee (1970) found a similar incidence of amnesia when scopolamine was given on its own. These and other early studies established that scopolamine on its own was associated with amnesia and was more potent in its effects on memory than atropine. This is consistent with a rigorous study by Domino and Corssen (1967) who compared equimolar doses of atropine and scopolamine and found that atropine showed less central effects than scopolamine and also that the methylated derivative of scopolamine, methscopolamine, showed no demonstrable central effects. The latter observation has been exploited in later studies where it has been shown that methscopolamine is devoid of effects on memory. This suggests that the effects of scopolamine on memory are exerted centrally.

More recent experimental studies designed to investigate further the nature of the effects of anticholinergic drugs on memory are based on these early experimental studies. Therefore scopolamine has usually been the anticholinergic drug investigated and it has been traditionally given parenterally in the same way as it is used for pre-medication. It is however quite effectively absorbed when given by the oral route, and is taken this way for the treatment of motion sickness.

Safer and Allen (1971) carried out extensive studies on the effects of various doses of scopolamine on human behaviour, including its effect on memory. They made two important findings which have been supported in other studies. Firstly, scopolamine in a dose of 10 μg/kg given intravenously only mildly impaired registration of new information or short-term memory measured by immediate recall on a digit span task, but performance after a 20-second delay was grossly impaired. They observed that this effect on memory was most prominent between 90 and 150 minutes after administration of the drug. The second finding was that scopolamine in doses of 4 and 8 μg/kg given by the same route did not affect memory for picture sorting and paired associated learning tasks memorized 30 minutes before drug administration. Retention of this information was unaffected during and following the expected time course of drug effect.

The finding that scopolamine has little effect on short-term memory as measured by digit span is supported by a study by Drachman and Leavitt (1974) who found intact digit span following a 1 mg dose of scopolamine given subcutaneously. Ghoneim and Mewaldt (1975) also found intact digit span, using a dose of 8 μg/kg given intramuscularly. The Brown-Peterson test, a standard procedure for testing the recall trigrams, has been used by Caine et al. (1981) to investigate the effects of scopolamine. Immediate recall was unaffected but delayed recall after 3–18 seconds was impaired, when rehearsal was prevented. Crow and Grove-White (1973) found that scopolamine in a fixed dose of 0.4 mg administered by intravenous injection impaired memory for a free-recall word list. The results were analysed by order of presentation of words within the ten-word lists. In the control condition the last three words in the list were better recalled than earlier items. This better performance on the last few words in the list, or recency effect, has been attributed to short-term memory although this has been recently challenged. The impairment in subjects' performance after scopolamine did not include performance on this portion of the recall curve, often attributed to short-term memory, but fell evenly on those parts of the curve attributed to long-term storage. In conclusion, despite disagreement about the significance of the effects of scopolamine on the free-recall paradigm, there is agreement that primary or short-term memory dealing with retaining small amounts of information for brief periods of time is intact after a dose of scopolamine which affects storage in long-term memory.

However, Jones et al. (1979) have carried out a study which may cast some doubt on the notion that short-term memory structures are inevitably intact following scopolamine. This study is of additional interest because only a modest oral dose of scopolamine (0.3 mg) was used, typical of the normal therapeutic dosage used in the treatment of motion sickness. They used an auditory digit span task requiring the recall of nine-digit strings in serial order. They found that the short-term retention of digits was impaired and that the locus of the effect was on the early items in the serial list, while performance on the final items was intact. The experimenters reasoned that performance on these early list items is generally considered to rely on short-term memory, and therefore scopolamine appears to influence the operation of this store. The final list items, where retention is intact following scopolamine, are thought to be under the control of pre-categorical acoustic storage which is envisaged as an acoustic buffer system, analogous to Sperling's visual buffer system. Therefore the mode of action of scopolamine may be interpreted to be task dependent, and it is dangerous to infer the mechanism of action of a drug from individual tasks. Rather, drug studies should be interpreted within a flexible theoretical framework.

Clearly there is evidence that scopolamine does leave intact some kind of primary memory structure; knowledge of drug effects should make a contribution to the definition of that structure. Several studies have supported Safer and Allen's original finding that scopolamine does not affect retention of material learned prior to drug administration. Ghoneim and Mewaldt (1977) and Petersen (1977) both presented word lists to subjects before and after administration of scopolamine and found that retention of the first list tested after scopolamine administration was intact, whereas performance on the second list presented and tested under the influence of the drug was grossly impaired. Ghoneim and Mewaldt used a dose of 8 μg/kg and tested retention by free recall and recognition. Petersen tested only by free recall but used a range of doses: 5, 8 and 10 μg/kg of scopolamine. In this study, although the result was not statistically significant, there appeared to be a trend of impaired recall with the highest dose. Petersen's study also provided additional results which were interpreted as consistent with intact retrieval. Four acquisition trials of word lists were given and subjects' recall was retested at various times up to twenty-four hours after drug. To assess the effects of the drug on recall independently of initial acquisition, a difference score was calculated which was used as an index of amount of material forgotten. It was found that scopolamine did not affect this measure. However, this study should be cautiously interpreted because the pharmacokinetics of scopolamine appear to have been overlooked.

The half-life of scopolamine has been found to be about seven hours and it was mentioned earlier that Safer and Allen found maximum drug effects on memory between 90 and 150 minutes after intravenous administration of the drug. In Petersen's study, certainly at the later time points, subjects would not have been tested under the influence of the drug.

On the basis of these experiments, most workers have postulated that scopolamine affects the acquisition but not the retrieval of information. Acquisition involves several stages, the initial registration, processing (encoding) and storage. Many workers have hypothesized that the locus of drug effect is on the transfer of information from short-term to long-term memory.

It has been suggested that scopolamine may also affect coding (encoding) processes but this has not yet been examined systematically. Ghoneim and Mewaldt (1975) tested recall of categorized and non-categorized words. They found that whereas subjects normally show significantly better recall performance on categorized rather than non-categorized words, the scopolamine-treated group did not use categorization effectively to improve recall. Categorization requires semantic coding and an effect of scopolamine on coding is a possibility. However, a retrieval difficulty could equally account for these results. In fact these findings are difficult to interpret as the overall low level of performance by the scopolamine group could have created a floor effect. Similarly Caine et al. (1981) observed that subjects treated with scopolamine were less able to distinguish high imagery words from low imagery words in a recall test with selective reminding. This study is equally open to various interpretations: Drachman and Leavitt (1974) and more recently Caine et al. (1981) suggest that scopolamine also has an effect on retrieval processes. In these studies the experimental task involved subjects naming as many words which began with a designated letter or fell into a certain category as they could in a given time. Scopolamine impaired performance on this type of task, which has been used to assess semantic memory. Therefore it appears a reasonable assumption that scopolamine affects retrieval processes involved in semantic memory, although further investigation is required. In this study, Drachman and Leavitt questioned the validity of the retrieval by category tests as they observed that drug-treated subjects tended to shift category during testing and often retrieved items from a different category after a brief time had elapsed.

The findings of Caine *et al.* (1981) are of further interest as they suggest that scopolamine may also affect retrieval from episodic memory. These researchers found that on a selective reminding task, learning deficits were mainly due to inconsistent recall of words that were previously remembered. Following scopolamine, subjects often repeated an item spontaneously for two or more trials before forgetting it. After being prompted, they would again recall the word several times, only to lose it again. Caine *et al.* also cite data from the study of Ghoneim and Mewaldt (1975) to support a drug effect on retrieval from episodic memory. In this study there was some apparent reversal of drug-induced forgetting with retention testing by recognition. However, a high level of performance on the recognition task by the placebo group may have created a ceiling effect. In any event, before the mechanism of action of scopolamine is ascribed to an effect on retrieval mechanisms, these findings need further investigation as there are methodological problems in separating drug effects on acquisition and retrieval.

One method of approaching the problem of separating drug effects on acquisition and retrieval is carefully to equate levels of original learning, perhaps by giving the scopolamine-treated subjects more exposure to the task. However, this type of drug study has not yet been carried out. The effects of scopolamine have usually been examined on verbal material presented auditorily, rather than visually; visual presentation of objects, pictures or non-verbal material has been little investigated. The effects of scopolamine on non-verbal visual material have been investigated by Ghoneim and Mewaldt (1975). They used a dose of 0.6 mg/70 kg intramuscularly and failed to obtain a drug effect on visual recognition of geometric shapes, but a ceiling effect may have contributed to this observation. Caine *et al.* (1981) used a similar dose of scopolamine (0.6–0.8 mg given intravenously) and used recall to test memory for patterns consisting of matrices of black and white squares. In this preliminary study, they found substantial drug effects.

In summary, there is evidence that anticholinergic drugs impair the operation of long-term memory, while not affecting a short-term memory system. On the basis of intact retention of material learned prior to drug administration, it has been argued that anticholinergic drugs impair acquisition but not retrieval. However, further studies are required in order to evaluate drug effects on retrieval from episodic memory. Retrieval from semantic memory does appear to be impaired. It is not known which aspect of acquisition of information is impaired by anticholinergic drugs. It has been hypothesized that coding or a transfer step from short-term to long-term memory may be involved. However, impairment of attention has also been put forward as a possible mechanism of action. Both Petersen (1977) and Ghoneim and Mewaldt (1977) have suggested that observed effects on memory function may be accounted for by an effect on attention. Ghoneim and Mewaldt found that subjects had difficulty in concentrating on tasks and reported that there was a tendency for their minds to wander. Drachman and Leavitt (1974) similarly noted apparent lapses of attention when subjects tended to shift category in a retrieval by category from semantic memory task. Caine *et al.* (1981) used a large battery of memory and non-memory tasks and found that the drug increased reaction time when subjects attended to acoustic signals in a vigilance task. Also to be considered are data on the effects of cholinergic drugs on attention, which are independent of the literature of drug effects on memory. Warburton (1979) has carried out a series of studies which suggest that attention is affected in vigilance tasks. Earlier studies by Calloway described by Warburton found effects of scopolamine on attention and suggested that the drug may affect selective attention, resulting in a broadening of attention with a reduced ability to filter out irrelevant stimuli. A drug effect on attention could account for all the effects on memory discussed above.

Traditionally, attentional processes have been considered separately from memory mechanisms by psychologists, but increasingly it is being acknowledged that as attention has a fundamental role in both input and retrieval of information, this may be an artificial exercise. In the same way that drug studies may help define memory structures, for example a primary memory structure, they may also help conceptualize the interaction of the various information processing structures which are brought to bear in the complex feat of memorizing. Anticholinergic drugs may have several effects on multiple processes involved in memory. There is strong physiological and biochemical evidence that parts of the limbic system, notably the hippocampus and the ascending reticular activating system, which itself has an input to the hippocampus, are major cholinergic systems. These areas appear to play an important role in memory in animals. It is interesting that recent studies suggest that lesions in the hippocampus may interfere with memory by impairing attention. However, physiologically it is likely that scopolamine affects several systems in the brain, as most brain areas contain significant numbers of muscarinic cholinergic receptors. Moreover other neurotransmitter systems, particularly noradrenergic pathways, have been implicated in both memory and attention. Drachman (1977) found that the effects of scopolamine could partly be reversed by physostigmine but not by amphetamine despite an improvement in alertness; this is consistent with an effect on cholinergic rather than noradrenergic mechanisms. However, the site of action of anticholinergic drugs is far from clear. It does seem likely that drug effects are the result of an action in the brain rather than a peripheral one. Caine *et al.* (1981) and Drachman and Leavitt (1974) found the peripherally acting anticholinergic drug methscopolamine to be devoid of effects on memory. However, not all studies have employed methscopolamine to control for peripheral effects. Drug effects on vision are particularly relevant, as anticholinergic drugs can increase pupil size and reduce the power of accommodation. Perceptual changes could account for some observed drug effects, particularly in attentional tasks. Safer and Allen (1971) found that there was some separation in the development of the peripheral effects and effects on memory and this could be exploited in designing drug studies. Whereas effects on memory reach their peak between 90 and 150 minutes following an intravenous dose of 10 μg/kg, effects on the eye are at maximum intensity after this.

In conclusion, scopolamine binds effectively to muscarinic receptors in the brain and it is usually assumed reasonably that this is the primary locus of action. What is still far from clear is where these receptors are and whether they are directly concerned with classical memory processes, e.g. storage and retrieval of information.

Cholinergic drugs   If drugs that antagonize muscarinic cholinergic receptors impair memory, it is rational to hypothesize that drugs which facilitate transmission at these receptors might improve memory. Deutsch and Rogers (1979) found that the anticholinesterase drugs (i.e. drugs which inhibit the breakdown of ACh) diisopropyl fluorophosphate (DFP) or physostigmine given after training could improve memory for a discrimination habit in rats, but this was dependent on the age of the memory at the time of drug treatment. For example, the drugs had no effect on a three-day habit, impaired memory of a seven- and fourteen-day habit and only facilitated memory at twenty-one days after training, when control animals showed forgetting. On the basis of these and other studies Deutsch argued that weak memories are faciliated by anticholinesterase drugs whereas strong memories are blocked, independent of whether memory strength is induced by age of memory, amount of training or habit difficulty.

Few studies have been carried out in man to investigate the effects of cholinergic drugs on memory. Partly this is due to problems with the adverse side-effects, short duration of action and lack of selectivity of these drugs for muscarinic receptors. Physostigmine, an anticholinesterase drug which readily crosses the blood-brain barrier, can cause undesirable central effects including a type of 'acute depression'. Peripheral side-effects which are troublesome include sweating and increased gut motility. Cardiovascular effects of bradycardia, and perhaps paradoxically a small increase in blood pressure, also occur and this means that subjects must undergo a rigorous medical check-up to screen for cardiovascular complaints. In healthy subjects peripheral, unwanted effects appear to be contained by pre-treatment with methscopolamine. However, central effects of depressed mood still remain and can be very unpleasant in some individuals. Happily, these wear off very quickly. The half-life of physostigmine is not known accurately, but it has been estimated to be only about thirty minutes, and this makes it difficult to design experiments.

Of course, anticholinesterase drugs facilitate transmission at both muscarinic and nicotinic receptors. This is also the case with the centrally acting agonists like arecoline which seem equally to have unpleasant side-effects, although perhaps a longer duration of action. Choline is possibly a more selective agonist for muscarinic receptors but its effects are weak and the exact mechanism of action is not clear.

Drachman (1977) found that a dose of 1 mg of physostigmine given subcutaneously reduced the impairment of memory produced by scopolamine. In an earlier study by Drachman and Leavitt (1974) it appeared that this dose of physostigmine on its own slightly improved memory on free recall of words, whereas a 2 mg dose impaired memory. However, these studies are difficult to interpret as long test batteries were used; it is therefore likely that subjects were not under the influence of physostigmine throughout. Other workers, including Davis et al. (1976), have found that 2–3 mg doses of physostigmine impair memory, and depress mood. In a more recent study, Davis et al. (1978) administered a 1 mg dose of physostigmine by slow infusion over a period of sixty minutes. Memory tests used included digit span and free recall of word lists which were presented before and after drug administration. Physostigmine did not affect digit span but improved recall of word lists presented during the drug infusion. It also improved recall of material learnt before drug administration. This was not significant eighteen minutes after the beginning of the infusion but reached significance ten minutes after the infusion stopped. Because of the uncertainty about the pharmacokinetics of physostigmine it is not clear whether there are higher plasma levels of drug at the later time. It is also possible that drug effects on retrieval are dependent on the strength of the memory trace, as in animal studies.

Davis *et al.* (1978) also found marked variability in the effects of physostigmine on memory and speculated that improvement may be correlated with a subject's baseline level of central cholinergic activity or ability. Subjects were pre-selected in their study to maximize the likelihood of improvement in memory function. High-ability subjects were excluded and it was not possible to examine whether drug effects depended on baseline cognitive functioning. In a study by Liljequist and Mattila (1979) this appeared to be the case. These workers examined the effects of physostigmine on memory function in chess players of graded ability. The tasks used consisted of problematic chess positions, shown to the subject on pictures. Percentage of correct positions of the chessman recalled was used to assess memory. Physostigmine impaired the performance of good players but improved performance when baseline performance was low. Although it appears from this study that subject variables were important determinants of drug effects, it is difficult to define these variables. There is no information on other aspects of memory ability in the chess players. It is likely that the players had to realize the strategic significance of the set of chessmen and use previously stored information in order to perform well on the task.

Sitaram *et al.* (1978) found that a 4 mg dose of arecoline given subcutaneously significantly enhanced serial learning of lists of categorized words. A similar improvement followed a 10 g oral dose of choline. The degree of improvement produced by the drugs was inversely proportional to a subject's performance on placebo. 'Poor performers' appeared to be more improved by drug. Other groups of workers have not been able to demonstrate an improvement in memory with choline. Mohs and Davis (1980) evaluated the effects of choline in subjects who had taken part in their earlier study of physostigmine.

They found that choline had no significant effect on average performance, either on acquisition or storage. However, the subjects who had
improved most when given physostigmine tended to show slight
improvement after choline. These results suggest that choline does
not have substantial effects on memory and, indeed, it appears to be
only a weak pharmacological agonist. They also reinforce the idea
that subject variables are important determinants of drug effects.

The hippocampus contains significant numbers of nicotinic as well
as muscarinic receptors and there has also been interest in the effects
of nicotine which stimulates nicotinic receptors relatively selectively.
In most studies, nicotine has been given as a cigarette to investigate
the effects of smoking on behaviour. In a similar way to physostigmine, nicotine has been associated with both improvements and
impairments in memory function. For example, Andersson (1974)
studied learning of nonsense syllables in habitual smokers in a smoking and non-smoking session. One single cigarette was smoked and
this contained 2.1 mg of nicotine. Immediately following the cigarette there was a decrease in the number of correct responses, but a
test of recall forty minutes after the end of the learning period showed
that retention was better in the smoking condition. These results were
interpreted in terms of a theory postulating a relationship between
arousal level and consolidation of memory. According to this theory,
the impairment in learning arises as a consequence of increased
arousal. High arousal at the time of learning is assumed to intensify
the consolidation process producing a better long-term memory but a
less available short-term trace. These effects on memory are not
specific to nicotine. The same kind of relationship between arousal
and memory has been demonstrated with white noise as the arousing
stimulus. Indeed, it is not clear whether nicotine was the stimulus in
Andersson's study, as a dummy nicotine-free cigarette was not used in
the control condition.

Thus, it does seem possible to improve memory by the use of cholinergic drugs. Although few studies have been carried out, physostigmine appears, despite other limitations, to be more effective than
cholinergic agonists acting on receptors. It is difficult to say why this
might be. One factor to take into consideration is that memory may
depend on phasic activity in the brain and therefore 'amplification of
the signal' may be more appropriate than indiscriminate stimulation
of receptors. In obtaining an improvement in memory, several other
variables may be important. These include dose of the drug, subject

variables and possibly strength of memory trace. Perhaps this is not really surprising. In normal individuals it is reasonable to suppose that transmitter function at cholinergic receptors in the brain is usually optimal. Moreover, cholinergic receptors, particularly nicotinic ones, are susceptible to desensitization and block in functioning if ACh levels are high. However, the suggestion of improved memory, at least under some circumstances, has encouraging implications for clinical studies and these are discussed in a later section of this chapter. Considered together, the experimental results suggest that boosting transmitter function at cholinergic receptors in the brain may facilitate both acquisition and retrieval of information in long-term memory, and these findings are consistent with those from the studies on scopolamine. As physostigmine antagonizes the effects of scopolamine on memory it appears that at least some of its memory-enhancing effects are attributable to an action on muscarinic receptors. However, nicotine itself also has effects on memory and therefore stimulation of nicotinic receptors may contribute to some of the observed effects. Most studies of nicotine have been carried out within a different theoretical framework to that used in studies of physostigmine. It is interesting that arousal and attentional mechanisms have been invoked to explain the effects of nicotine and this is also analogous to the scopolamine literature.

Drugs affecting brain catecholamines

There are numerous catecholamine systems in the brain. The ascending noradrenergic innervation to the limbic forebrain has been strongly associated with attention in animal studies. It has also been shown that centrally administered noradrenaline, isoprenaline and dopamine given post-training can improve retention whereas the catecholamine antagonists propranolol and diethyldithiocarbamate can impair both acquisition and retention. Amphetamine, administered systemically, also improves retention but it appears that at least some of its effects are peripheral and possibly mediated by catecholamine systems involved in arousal. As with manipulation of the cholinergic system, drug responses in animals depend on a number of variables. In the case of drugs affecting catecholamine systems, task and dose are particularly important. For example, the same post-training dose of *d*-amphetamine or adrenaline can facilitate retention of avoidance behaviour with low footshock or after extensive pre-training but impair retention after high footshock or minimal pre-training. It is generally believed that the state of arousal of the animal interacts with a certain dose of drug to determine performance. Similarly, in man it is well known that performance enhancing effects of stimulant drugs given before testing are seen particularly when a task is physically tiring or intellectually undemanding. In simple psychomotor tests like routine mental arithmetic and cancellation, amphetamine often improves performance. However, in more intellectually demanding tasks amphetamine does not improve performance unless it is already impaired, by sleep deprivation, for example. Few studies have been carried out to examine the effects of these drugs specifically on memory. Mewaldt and Ghoneim (1979) investigated the effects of meth-amphetamine on memory and found that the drug did not affect free recall of words presented before drug injection. There was a small improvement in words learned after injection. However, this was accompanied by a large increase in incorrect responding. A study by Hurst *et al.* (1969) using a paired associate learning task showed a small improvement in retention with *d*-amphetamine when the drug was given before learning, but not when it was given after learning. However, these facilitatory effects of amphetamine on paired associate learning have not been supported in other studies. Perhaps discrepancies in the literature may be accounted for by differences in the age of the subjects. Several studies have been carried out using normal children as subjects. This is because of the apparent clinical benefits of stimulant drugs on the behaviour and performance of hyperkinetic children. In normal pre-pubertal boys, Rapoport *et al.* (1978) found that amphetamine facilitated word list recall. It also improved vigilance on a continuous performance test and similar effects have been demonstrated in hyperkinetic children. However, studies in normal adults have found impaired memory and attention with similar doses of stimulant drugs. In a recent study, Wetzel *et al.* (1981) investigated three dose levels of methylphenidate on various memory tasks, and concluded that the drug impaired performance by disrupting attention during learning.

It appears that stimulant drugs can improve performance including memory, but this is very dependent on task and subject variables. It might occur most reliably when subjects are performing suboptimally, for a variety of reasons. In man, improvement in memory only occurs when the drugs are administered before learning. Drug effects may therefore be exerted primarily on acquisition. However, effects on retrieval have been little investigated in man. Under conditions where performance is assumed to be optimal, both impairment in memory and attention has usually been observed. The mechanism of action of stimulant drugs is far from clear. Animal studies demonstrate that stimulant drugs can facilitate release of noradrenaline and dopamine, and also act as agonists at various catecholamine receptors in the brain and in the peripheral nervous system. Drugs that will cross the blood-brain barrier and selectively stimulate catecholamine receptors are in general not available for human experimental studies. L-dopa crosses the blood-brain barrier and may show some selectivity for facilitating dopaminergic transmission. However, effects on memory have only been investigated in patient groups and in preliminary studies effects have not been reliably demonstrated. Some selective antagonists are available and studies of these drugs will help to clarify mechanisms. Some studies of β-blocking drugs have been carried out, particularly with propranolol. Propranolol blocks β receptors both in the brain and in the periphery. It has been shown to have little if any effect on a number of tasks, including some with a memory component, although prolongation of simple reaction time and slight sedative effects have been demonstrated.

On balance it appears from experimental studies that manipulation of catecholamine systems does not offer much promise for improving memory in patients. However, in Korsakoff's syndrome this approach has met with some success and this will be detailed in a later section.

Peptides

Adrenocorticotrophic hormone (ACTH) Animal studies of $ACTH_{1-39}$ or the fragment $ACTH_{4-10}$ suggest that some central effects of these drugs on attention are rather similar to those produced by depletion of forebrain noradrenaline and have been described as a failure to ignore irrelevant stimuli. Effects on memory have also been observed and these appear to occur under similar conditions to those reported with amphetamine. Thus ACTH given post-training can facilitate retention of passive avoidance with low intensity footshock, but impairs retention if high intensity footshock has been used in training. ACTH may, like amphetamine, improve memory by increasing arousal and there is evidence that a peripheral mechanism may also be involved.

There have been a few studies of $ACTH_{4-10}$ in man. An experiment by Miller *et al.* (1976) is fairly representative, both of the type of experimental protocol and of the findings obtained in these studies. Miller and his colleagues investigated the effects of a 30 mg dose of $ACTH_{4-10}$ on a continuous performance test and various memory tasks. The stimuli in the continuous performance test were arranged in blocks, where the ratio of relevant stimuli to irrelevant stimuli changed. Improved performance on this task was observed but effects were small and only seen during the first time the stimulus ratio was changed. The authors interpreted this as an effect on attention, occurring when subjects were developing new expectancies and therefore the attentional demand of the task was greatest. They also reasoned that the results could not be accounted for by a general activating effect producing an indiscriminate increase in response which can be observed with amphetamine. This conclusion was based on the finding that not only were errors of omission significantly reduced but there were also fewer errors of commission. Memory quotient on the Wechsler memory scale was also improved although effects were not seen consistently across all subtests. It appeared that these results could also be explained on an attentional basis as the tasks which required immediate, focused attention such as digit span were improved but other tasks, including memory for a prose passage, were not. Although it might be argued from the data on digit span that ACTH can improve short-term memory, these findings have not been supported by the results of other short-term memory tasks including the Brown-Peterson paradigm, and memory for short sequences of letters presented visually has been reported to be impaired. An impairment in attention would be consistent with the animal literature. Clearly the nature of the effects of ACTH in man are still unclear. In particular the interesting suggestion that effects of ACTH on attention may be more specific than those of stimulant drugs needs further investigation.

Vasopressin   Arginine-8-vasopressin and lysine-8-vasopressin have similar effects to ACTH in animals except that vasopressin's effects on behaviour are of longer duration and can last for several days. In addition rats with reduced vasopressin in the brain induced by intraventricular administration of antiserum to arginine-8-vasopressin show impaired retention. These findings and also the apparent long duration of action of the drug have raised hopes that it may be useful in the treatment of various memory disorders. Clinical studies on patients are referred to later but to date there appear to have been no well-controlled experimental studies in normal individuals.

Benzodiazepines

The effects of various benzodiazepines on psychomotor function in man have been investigated in numerous studies, some of which have included tests of memory in the experimental protocol. These drugs usually impair performance, including memory function, although tolerance often develops with chronic treatment. Occasionally small improvements in performance have been observed and this has been accounted for by the anxiety-reducing properties of these drugs. Of particular interest are a series of studies by Ghoneim and Mewaldt. These workers have compared the effects of diazepam on memory with those of scopolamine. In 1975 Ghoneim and Mewaldt reported that diazepam, like scopolamine, did not affect digit span, nor did the drugs impair recall of information which had been learned before drug administration. However, administered before learning both drugs impaired the acquisition of lists of words. In a later study, Ghoneim and Mewaldt (1977) confirmed these findings and concluded that diazepam and scopolamine have similar effects on memory. They did observe small differences in drug effects but thought that these could be accounted for by differences in duration of drug action. An additional observation was that while physostigmine antagonized most of the memory deficits induced by scopolamine, it did not antagonize the effects of diazepam.

The finding that these drugs have similar effects is supported by a study by Jones *et al.* (1979) described previously. They found that retention of digit strings was impaired to an equivalent degree and locus with oral doses of 5 mg of diazepam and 0.3 mg of scopolamine, and they concluded that both drugs impair primary memory. Barnett *et al.* (1980) used a similar paradigm and obtained interesting data. Their subjects were first divided into a high- and low-anxiety group after a test of state of anxiety. In accord with the result of Jones *et al.* (1979) the performance of the low-anxiety group deteriorated with a 5 mg dose of diazepam, although this difference was not significant. However, diazepam significantly improved performance of the high-anxiety group. In a recent study Ghoneim *et al.* (1981) found that when diazepam was administered chronically for three weeks, effects on memory diminished.

In conclusion, apart perhaps from the ability of diazepam to improve performance in some subjects, and development of tolerance to effects on memory, the effects of diazepam and scopolamine appear similar. However, we have as yet no information on the effects of chronic treatment with scopolamine or the dependence of drug action on baseline anxiety level. Further investigation is needed to compare drug effects in more detail.

However, it may be that the pattern of memory deficit is essentially common to several drugs which impair memory. Yet the finding that the effects of scopolamine but not diazepam are reversed by physostigmine indicates that the drugs are acting by different mechanisms. Benzodiazepines facilitate transmission at GABA receptors in the brain and these are found in all areas which have been implicated in memory function, including the hippocampus.

Miscellaneous drugs

There have been a few reports of other drugs improving memory. For example, Dimond and Brouwers (1976) suggested that piracetam may have memory enhancing effects in normal volunteers. Both the pharmacological properties of this drug and its effects on memory need further investigation.

A large number of drugs have been reported to impair performance on memory tests. These include barbiturates, phenothiazines, tricyclic antidepressants, alcohol, marijuana and the lithium ion. However, few studies have been carried out to investigate the nature of the effects on memory function. More importantly these studies have often been carried out in isolation with no attempt to make comparisons with reference compounds, for example anticholinergic drugs. Crow *et al.* (1976) carried out a preliminary study of various doses of chlorpromazine and amylobarbitone and compared their effects to those of scopolamine. They found that whereas scopolamine impaired memory on verbal learning but did not affect performance on a scanning task, chlorpromazine in a dose which affected memory also reduced performance on the scanning task. No significant effects of amylobarbitone on memory occurred with a drug dose which affected scanning. However, in this study a 5 mg dose of diazepam had no effects on memory. This illustrates the point that for valid drug comparison several doses of drugs and various memory paradigms need to be employed. Tricyclic antidepressants, for example imipramine, appear to have similar effects to anticholinergic drugs on memory. Probably this is because most of these drugs have marked antimuscarinic properties. Lithium, which is used in the treatment of mood disorder, has also been reported to impair memory, at least after chronic treatment. In addition, physostigmine has been found to significantly improve performance on the full scale IQ of the Wechsler Adult Intelligence Scale when given in conjunction with lithium in patients with manic depressive illness. Therefore, although lithium can impair memory it may also potentiate the effects of physostigmine and promote an improvement in cognitive function under some circumstances. These findings with lithium deserve further investigation. Potentiation of the effects of physostigmine might be very useful clinically.

Clinical investigations

Clinical disorders of memory

Neuropsychological studies of memory disorder have provided support for constructs of multiple memory structures. Selective impairment of different memory systems has been observed in patients with focal brain pathology and lesions. Also histological and biochemical studies of the brain in these conditions have provided clues about possible neurotransmitter substrates of memory mechanisms, with pharmacological implications.

Memory disorder is found in a variety of conditions: in the Korsakoff syndrome, following herpes simplex encephalitis, and after temporal lobectomy. It is also seen in several degenerative diseases including Alzheimer's disease and Huntington's chorea. Trauma including stroke and electro-convulsive therapy (ECT) can also give rise to memory disorder and normal old age also appears to be associated with memory deficits, at least in some individuals. All these memory disorders have been investigated in some detail but Korsakoff's syndrome and patients with temporal lobe damage have received most attention. There is little information available about memory disorders following herpes simplex encephalitis, where survivors are rare. Also we have only limited knowledge of the memory disorder of Alzheimer's disease because studies have generally been carried out in the later stages of the disease when memory deficits are confounded by other cognitive defects, making interpretation difficult.

Although there is a substantial body of data on some individual disorders, it is difficult to make comparisons between the various aetiologies. This is because different neuropsychological methodologies have often been used for patient groups and also because types of patient have not always been rigorously defined. Sometimes this is difficult to do. For example in Korsakoff's syndrome the pathology has been found not to be homogeneous in patients and to arrange for follow-up autopsy studies on patients who have been tested in life is not always practicable.

Several studies of amnesic patients have assumed a distinction between short-time and long-term memory and investigated whether short-term memory is intact. There is agreement that memory span is intact in most patients, whether they are suffering from temporal lobe damage, are post-encephalitic or have Korsakoff's syndrome.

Baddeley and Warrington (1970) have investigated immediate free recall of word lists in amnesic patients with the above range of clinical conditions. In these studies performance showed a gross impairment of retention of earlier items in the list, generally assumed to depend on long-term memory, while performance was not impaired on the most recent items, recall of which is often attributed to short-term memory. Similarly Baddeley and Warrington found patients unimpaired on the Brown-Peterson task of trigram recall, a task purported to rely on short-term memory.

On the basis of these and other studies Weiskrantz and Warrington (1976) have postulated that the memory defect is a retrieval difficulty. Two groups of findings led to this conclusion. Firstly patients were asked to remember lists of words on a series of occasions and it was noted that on a particular occasion not only did subjects have difficulty in remembering words that had just been presented to them but they made numerous mistakes or intrusion errors, many of which were words that had been presented to them in an earlier session. This suggested that patients were capable of acquiring and storing significant amounts of information. Secondly, in another series of experiments, it was found that memory for words or pictures, although defective under free recall or recognition conditions, could be enhanced to almost normal levels when subjects were cued with a fragment of the original item. Initially these results were interpreted to be consistent with a proactive interference hypothesis; this suggests that poor memory is not due to an initial weak memory trace but is caused by increased sensitivity to the interfering effects of other irrelevant traces. It was argued that cues were helpful by constraining inappropriate responses. Further experiments have demonstrated that a simple interference hypothesis is not adequate to explain the memory deficits of these patients.

Recently Weiskrantz (1978) and others have advanced a hypothesis which is consistent with data from the above experiments and also takes into account findings that perceptual and motor learning is intact in these patients. It is suggested that amnesic patients can acquire information but normally do not have access to the products of learning. However, when a task gives the patient an opportunity to show learning without demanding him to commit himself to where the information originated, learning is intact. For example in the cueing studies the subject is only required to submit a response to fit with the stimulus and does not need to be aware of whether he has or has not seen that item before. This is an attractive hypothesis, but it is not supported by all workers and even the basic assumption of intact acquisition has been questioned, on two lines of evidence. Briefly, studies by a group in Boston led by Butters (Butters and Cermak, 1976) have found that Korsakoff patients are poorer at the Brown-Peterson task than controls, although it should be pointed out that they organized the task in a slightly different way from Baddeley and his co-workers. Secondly, the same group has reported that Korsakoff patients show impaired coding and suggest that this results in a weak memory trace. The group also suggests that improved performance by cueing acts only to reinforce this initial weak memory trace. Contrary to this interpretation is the fact that Weiskrantz and Warrington's patients were impaired in recognition, i.e. the whole word did not afford as good a cue as the first three letters. Baddeley (1979) has since suggested that one reason for discrepancies between the results of the two groups is that their own patients were highly selected to have intact cognition apart from memory problems while the American studies took 'all-comers' with Korsakoff's syndrome, and therefore deficits they observed might be real but secondary to basic memory problems. In fact the British approach has been to study memory and its failure, using any patient who appears to show memory failure in a relatively pure form, whereas other studies have concentrated on describing Korsakoff's syndrome in its full clinical spectrum.

It is relevant to mention here that although there can be some overlap in brain areas damaged in the various conditions, this is not always the case. On the basis of pathological and neuropsychological data Squire (1982) has speculated that there might be two types of amnesia. The first type is purported to be due to damage to the diencephalon for example as in Korsakoff's syndrome and consists of a deficit in the initial coding of information. The second type is due to bilateral damage to the temporal lobes including the hippocampus and this is reflected in a deficit in post-coding processes involved in the consolidation of memory. This idea was originally put forward by Milner (1966) to describe H.M., a patient with damage to the temporal lobes. Squire would also include post-ECT patients in this category. Patients with Alzheimer's disease and post-encephalitics also have damage to the temporal lobes, particularly the hippocampus, but it is not clear whether they fall into a clear category. For example, patients with Alzheimer's disease have been shown to give intrusion errors and be aided by cueing while at the same time there is evidence for impaired acquisition of information and other cognitive dysfunction. Studies in the early stages of the disease are awaited with interest, as this group of patients is very numerous in contrast to the other patient groups, and knowledge of the nature of the cognitive deficit would help in rational psychopharmacological studies, with a view to the development of treatments for memory disorder in this condition.

Biochemical studies have been carried out in Korsakoff's syndrome and in Alzheimer's disease. In Korsakoff's syndrome thalamic lesions may be associated with monoamine containing neurones and decreased levels of 3-methoxy-4-hydroxphenyl glycol, the main metabolite of noradrenaline, have been found in the lumbar cerebro-spinal fluid of patients with Korsakoff's syndrome. Experiments on animals also suggest that noradrenaline plays a role in learning and memory. In Alzheimer's disease a large number of studies have demonstrated that the synthetic enzyme choline acetyltransferase, and the ability there-fore to synthesize acetylcholine, is deficient in the temporal lobes, particularly the hippocampus, in patients with this disorder. Other transmitters including GABA and the neuropeptide somatostatin may also be affected. The hippocampus and cholinergic mechanisms have been widely implicated in memory processes in animal studies.

Cholinergic drugs

Most studies of cholinergic drugs have been carried out in Alzheimer's disease or related conditions. Alzheimer's disease is fairly common and occurs in at least 5 per cent of people over the age of sixty-five, but much less frequently in younger people. Memory disorder is usually present in this condition, often in the early stages, and a cholinergic deficit is found, particularly in the hippocampal formation and temporal neocortex. However, Alzheimer's disease is a progressive degenerative disease and other symptoms, including progressive dementia, language disorder and apraxia, occur at a later stage and even sometimes in the early stages. In fact the brain tissue often degenerates very quickly and changes in other transmitter systems have now been described, although it appears that these may be secondary to the cholinergic deficits.

Smith and Swash (1978) and other workers have suggested that the memory disorder may be related to the cholinergic deficit. It was pointed out earlier that although memory deficits in various clinical conditions may be heterogeneous both between and within diagnostic groups, they seem to have common features. Briefly, it has been observed that some patients with Alzheimer's disease on memory testing make intrusion errors which appear rather similar to those observed in the amnesic syndrome by Warrington and Weiskrantz (1976). These workers drew attention to evidence that on the descriptive level animals with lesions of the hippocampus show perseveration of responses or strategies, i.e. give responses learned earlier which are no longer appropriate to a new learning situation. They suggested that these responses may be comparable with the cognitive interference seen in their amnesic patients. The physiology of disinhibited behaviour has been investigated in animals and it has been shown that interruption of cholinergic connections between the septum and hippocampus can produce disinhibited behaviour (as can other lesions and drug treatment). Several workers have supported this position and suggested an information-processing role for the hippocampus in enabling the organism to ignore or to filter out biologically irrelevant or redundant stimuli via a cholinergic mechanism.

It was these observations and the well-known findings that anticholinergic drugs impair memory in man and can mimic amnesic syndromes which suggested to us that damage to cholinergic pathways, possibly running to or from the hippocampus, could be an important factor in the memory disorder of early Alzheimer's disease and that it might be possible to improve memory by the use of cholinergic drugs. In most studies choline, in the form of a choline salt or purified lecithin preparation, has been administered. Lecithin (phosphatidyl choline) is a natural source of choline which is found in many foodstuffs including eggs and fish. On a normal diet plasma choline levels are usually maintained within narrow limits and quite large amounts of choline need to be administered to increase plasma levels significantly. Smith *et al.* (1978) carried out a double-blind crossover study where 9 g of choline were administered for two weeks. No drug effects were observed on a battery of memory tests. These included tests of free recall of word lists and recognition of visual material, including photographs. Recall of more meaningful material including memory for a name, address and shopping list was also employed.

A variety of other studies of choline given in various forms and for several time periods has failed to provide good evidence for an improvement in memory function. Originally it was thought that choline might act in analogous fashion to l-dopa on the dopamine system, making more ACh available in the brain. It was an attractive idea, as it also appeared that daily administration of choline might keep choline plasma levels high and give a sustained drug effect. However, biochemical and pharmacological studies now suggest that choline is a weak agonist at ACh receptors and may have no effect on ACh synthesis. Further, not surprisingly, there seems to be some homeostatic mechanism to maintain choline plasma levels. In patients we have found that plasma levels of choline tend to fall during chronic administration, and this has been confirmed by others. As described previously, there is some evidence that choline may have some slight beneficial effects on memory in normal volunteers. This may also be the case in patients with Alzheimer's disease, as there is an unconfirmed report that lecithin administration appears to potentiate the effects of physostigmine on memory. We have not observed improvement of memory in Alzheimer's disease with a 1 mg dose of physostigmine given subcutaneously using a similar test to that used in the choline study; however, intrusion errors of various kinds were reduced, and our patients were moderately demented. In a post-encephalitic patient with mild cognitive impairment, another group of researchers used the same dose of physostigmine and found that a reduction in extra-list intrusion errors was accompanied by improved performance on learning lists of words. In Alzheimer's disease physostigmine has also been reported to both reduce mistakes and improve performance. In these studies some of the patients were reported to have only mild memory and other problems, and physostigmine was given as an infusion. In a study by

Christie *et al.* (1981) significant improvement was seen on a picture recognition test with 0.375 mg of physostigmine administered intravenously over 30 minutes and also with 4 mg of arecholine. A trend towards improvement was also seen with 0.25 and 0.75 mg of physostigmine. Improvement of recognition with a similar physostigmine infusion has been reported by other workers who also found that the dose of physostigmine was very critical. High doses of the drug can cause impaired performance and the optimal dose to cause improvement in memory varies between individuals.

These results appear to be encouraging. However, further investigation is required. Firstly, more studies of the nature of the cognitive deficits in Alzheimer's disease are required, otherwise it is not possible to choose tests which seem likely to predict therapeutic benefits. The recognition tests referred to above were chosen from various others, including word lists, because the patients were able to perform at a reasonable level on them: this is consistent with other evidence that recognition memory for faces is relatively well preserved in patients with early Alzheimer's disease. Clearly, what is required are drug studies in patients with early disease using tests that the patient has particular difficulty with, provided that care is taken that the patient fully understands the instructions and a baseline performance can be established. Otherwise an improved performance with physostigmine might easily be accounted for by non-specific effects of the drug, perhaps on general arousal and not directly related to the core deficits in the condition. This would be consistent with the known facts that cholinergic neurones are very widely distributed in the brain and that performance in normal individuals can be enhanced with physostigmine.

In summary, clarification of the nature of the memory deficit in Alzheimer's disease will help in the planning of further drug studies. At the moment there are few guidelines to determine what the nature of the core disabilities might be as, unfortunately, much of the neuro-psychological literature does not differentiate between patients with different types of dementia. It is clear that selective attention in the input of information has been little investigated but there are indications that this may be impaired. On the basis of our preliminary studies and other observations, it would also seem that the role of selective attention in retrieval of information warrants further study. A further stumbling-block in the development of treatments is that the only drugs demonstrating effects, i.e. physostigmine and possibly arecholine, have only short biological half-lives. Thus, at the moment it appears that although cholinergic drugs are worthy of further study, full clinical trials of these agents are not warranted until more basic research has been carried out.

Drugs affecting brain catecholamines

As described previously, catecholamines have been implicated in the memory disorder occurring in Korsakoff's syndrome. McEntee and Mair (1980) tested three drugs which enhance catecholamine activity by different mechanisms, d-amphetamine, clonidine and methysergide, in this condition using a neuropsychological test battery. Only clonidine, 0.3 mg given orally for two weeks, was associated with a significant improvement in memory. Tests were chosen on the basis that they were similar or identical to tasks on which patients with Korsakoff's syndrome have been reported to perform significantly worse than normal controls. Clonidine caused an overall improvement of memory quotient on the Wechsler memory scale and this was accounted for by an improvement in memory passages and visual reproduction. Memory for a prose passage demonstrated a highly significant difference between clonidine and placebo. These preliminary data are very interesting, particularly as the drug did appear to show some selective effects, only improving memory deficits which occur in this condition. For example, digit span was not significantly improved. The mechanism of action of clonidine in the brain is not fully elucidated. It is an agonist at both presynaptic and postsynaptic α-receptors, and appears to interfere with learning in animals. On balance, its presynaptic effects appear to dominate, and it therefore acts by decreasing the release of noradrenaline.

Miscellaneous drugs

Several uncontrolled studies of vasopressin in various kinds of memory disorder are encouraging. However, controlled studies in Alzheimer's disease have failed to demonstrate any benefits. Similarly, $ACTH_{4-10}$, 30 mg subcutaneously, has been reported to improve mood and it appears to improve in patients with 'mild senile organic brain syndrome', but effects on memory have not been convincingly demonstrated.

There have been numerous clinical studies of a variety of other drugs in elderly patients with memory disorder. These include drugs claimed to improve cell metabolism, vasodilators and piracetam. The results of these preliminary studies are equivocal, except perhaps for hydergine which does seem to improve global functioning, particularly with respect to mood, alertness, and short-term memory. This drug was originally developed as a vasodilator but is now thought to act by improving brain cell metabolism. Although small improvements in cognitive functioning have been demonstrated in patients with Alzheimer's disease and other diagnoses, the role of hydergine in therapeutics is not yet established.

Conclusions

Inevitably this chapter has mainly discussed drugs affecting cholinergic synapses as the literature on drugs affecting other systems is sparse and not easy to interpret. It is difficult to make comparisons between the effects of the various types of drug, not only because of lack of data, but also because studies have often evolved quite separately and are therefore based on a different theoretical framework and experimental protocol. Despite these limitations there do appear to be some similarities in their final mode of action. It is clear that it is easier to impair memory with drugs than it is to improve it, at least in normal subjects. One reason for this is that drug effects on memory described so far may be exerted on attentional mechanisms, which are only one component in the memory process. Rational attempts to improve memory in patients have only just begun. However, the results from some studies do appear encouraging. Probably the effects of cholinergic drugs in Alzheimer's disease are most promising and this may be because attentional deficits are important in the memory disorder in this condition. It is certain that there is no 'magic bullet' to improve memory at the moment. However the idea that there is such a drug which may act on a yet undiscovered substrate in the brain and perhaps improve processing or storage is a very attractive notion and one which will continue to motivate research workers for the foreseeable future.

References

Andersson, K. (1974) Effects of cigarette smoking on learning and retention. *Psychopharmacologia 41*: 1–5.

Atkinson, R. C. and Shiffrin, R. M. (1971) The control of short-term memory. *Scientific American 225*: 82–90.

Baddeley, A. D. (1979) A minimal model and an interpretation. In L. Cermak (ed.) *Proceedings of the Memory and Amnesia Conference.* Hillsdale NJ: Erlbaum.

Baddeley, A. D. and Hitch, G. (1974) Working memory. In G. A. Bower (ed.) *The Psychology of Learning and Motivation.* Vol. 8. New York: Academic Press.

Baddeley, A. D. and Warrington, E. K. (1970) Amnesia and the distinction between long- and short-term memory. *Journal of Verbal Learning and Verbal Behaviour 9:* 176–89.

Barnett, D. B., Davies, A. T. and Desai, D. (1980) Differential effect of diazepam on short-term memory in high and low anxious subjects. *Proceedings of the British Pharmacological Society,* December.

Broadbent, D. E. (1958) *Perception and Communication.* London and New York: Pergamon.

Buschke, H. (1973) Selective reminding for analysis of memory and learning. *Journal of Verbal Learning and Verbal Behaviour 12*: 543–50.

Butters, N. and Cermak, L. (1976) Some analyses of amnesic syndromes in brain-damaged patients. In R. L. Isaacson and K. H. Pribram (eds) *Hippocampus.* Vol. 2. New York: Plenum.

Caine, E. D., Weingartner, H., Ludlow, C. L., Cudahy, E. A. and Wehry, S. (1981) Qualitative analysis of scopolamine-induced amnesia. *Psychopharmacology 74*: 74–80.

Christie, J. E., Shering, A., Ferguson, J. and Glen, A. I. M. (1981) Physostigmine and arecoline: effects of intravenous infusions in Alzheimer Presenile Dementia. *British Journal of Psychiatry 138*: 46–50.

Crow, T. J. and Grove-White, I. G. (1973) An analysis of the learning deficit following hyoscine administration to man. *British Journal of Pharmacology 49*: 322–7.

Crow, T. J., Grove-White, I. and Ross, D. G. (1976) The specificity of the action of hyoscine on human learning. *British Journal of Clinical Pharmacology 2*: 367–8.

Davis, K. L., Hollister, L. E., Overall, J., Johnson, A. and Train, K. (1976) Physostigmine: effects on cognition and affect in normal subjects. *Psychopharmacology 51*: 23–7.

Davis, K. L., Mohs, R. C., Tinklenberg, J. R., Pfefferbaum, A., Hollister, L. E. and Kopell, B. S. (1978) Physostigmine: improvement of long-term memory processes in normal humans. *Science 201*: 272–4.

Deutsch, J. A. and Rogers, J. B. (1979) Cholinergic excitability and memory: animal studies and their clinical implications. In K. L. Davis and P. A. Berger (eds) *Brain Acetylcholine and Neuropsychiatric Disease.* New York: Plenum.

Dimond, S. J. and Brouwers, E. Y. M. (1976) Increase in the power of memory in normal man through the use of drugs. *Psychopharmacology 49*: 307–9.

Domino, E. F. and Corssen, G. (1967) Central and peripheral effects of muscarinic cholinergic blocking agents in man. *Anaesthesiology 28*: 568–74.

Drachman, D. A. (1977) Memory and cognitive function in man. Does the cholinergic system have a specific role? *Neurology 27*: 783–90.

Drachman, D. A. and Leavitt, J. (1974) Human memory and the cholinergic system. *Archives of Neurology 30*: 113–21.

Ghoneim, M. M. and Mewaldt, S. P. (1975) Effects of diazepam and scopolamine on storage retrieval and organisational processes in memory. *Psychopharmacologia 44*: 257–62.

Ghoneim, M. M. and Mewaldt, S. P. (1977) Studies on human memory: the interactions of diazepam, scopolamine and physostigmine. *Psychopharmacology 52*: 1–6.

Ghoneim, M. M., Mewaldt, S. P., Berie, J. L. and Hinrichs, J. V. (1981) Memory and performance effects of single and 3 week administration of diazepam. *Psychopharmacology 73*: 147–51.

Hardy, T. K. and Wakely, D. (1962) The amnesic properties of hyoscine and atropine in pre-anaesthetic medication. *Anaesthesia 17*: 331–6.

Hurst, P. M., Radlow, R., Chubb, N. C. and Bagley, S. K. (1969) Effects of d-amphetamine on acquisition, persistence and recall. *American Journal of Psychology 82*: 307–19.

Jones, D. M., Jones, M. E. L., Lewis, M. J. and Spriggs, T. L. B. (1979) Drugs and human memory: effects of low doses of nitrazepam and hyoscine on retention. *British Journal of Clinical Pharmacology 7*: 479–83.

Liljequist, R. and Mattila, M. J. (1979) Effect of physostigmine and scopolamine on the memory functions of chess players. *Medical Biology 57*: 402–5.

McEntee, W. J. and Mair, R. G. (1980) Memory enhancement in Korsakoff's psychosis by clonidine. Further evidence for a noradrenergic deficit. *Annals of Neurology 7*: 466–70.

Mewaldt, S. P. and Ghoneim, M. M. (1979) The effects and interactions of scopolamine, physostigmine and methamphetamine on human memory. *Pharmacology, Biochemistry and Behavior 10*: 205–10.

Miller, L. H., Harris, L. C., van Riezen, H. and Kastin, A. J. (1976) Neuroheptapeptide influence on attention and memory in man. *Pharmacology, Biochemistry and Behavior 5*, Suppl. 1: 17–21.

Milner, B. (1966) Amnesia following operation on the temporal lobes. In C. W. M. Whitty and O. L. Zangwill (eds) *Amnesia*. London and Washington, DC.: Butterworths, pp. 109–33.

Mohs, R. C. and Davis, K. L. (1980) Choline chloride effects on memory: correlation with the effects of physostigmine. *Psychiatry Research 2*: 149–56.

Pandit, S. K. and Dundee, J. W. (1970) Pre-operative amnesia. *Anaesthesia 25*: 493–9.

Petersen, R. C. (1977) Scopolamine induced learning failures in man. *Psychopharmacology 52*: 283–9.

Rapoport, J. L., Zahn, T. P., Ludlow, C. and Mikkelsen, E. J. (1978) Dextro-amphetamine: cognitive and behavioral effects in normal prepubertal boys. *Science 199*: 560–3.

Safer, D. J. and Allen, R. P. (1971) The central effects of scopolamine in man. *Biological Psychiatry 3*: 347–55.

Sitaram, N., Weingartner, H. and Gillin, J. C. (1978) Human serial learning: enhancement with arecoline and impairment with scopolamine correlated with performance on placebo. *Science 201*: 274–6.

Smith, C. M. and Swash, M. (1978) Possible biochemical basis of memory disorder in Alzheimer's disease. *Annals of Neurology 3*: 471–3.

Smith, C. M. and Swash, M. (1979) Physostigmine in Alzheimer's disease. *Lancet i*: 42.

Smith, C. M., Swash, M., Exton-Smith, A. N., Phillips, M. J., Overstall, P. W., Piper, M. E. and Bailey, M. R. (1978) Choline in Alzheimer's disease. *Lancet ii*: 318.

Squire, L. R. (1982) The neuropsychology of human memory. In *Annual Review of Neuroscience 5*: 241–74.

Tulving, E. (1972) Episodic and semantic memory. In E. Tulving and W. Donaldson (eds) *Organization of Memory*. New York: Academic Press.

Warburton, D. M. (1979) Neurochemical basis of consciousness. In K. Brown and S. J. Cooper (eds) *Chemical Influences on Behaviour*. London: Academic Press.

Weiskrantz, L. (1978) A comparison of hippocampal pathology in man and animals. In Ciba Foundation's Symposium 58. *Functions of the Septo-Hippocampal System*. North Holland: Elsevier.

Weiskrantz, L. and Warrington, E. K. (1976) The problem of the amnesic syndrome in man and animals. In R. L. Isaacson and K. H. Pribram (eds) *Hippocampus*. Vol. 2. New York: Plenum.

Wetzel, C. D., Squire, L. R. and Janowsky, D. S. (1981) Methylphenidate impairs learning and memory in normal adults. *Behavioural and Neural Biology 31*: 413–24.

7 The use of drugs in psychiatry

P. E. Harrison-Read

Introduction

This chapter is about drug treatment of mental disorders, and will also deal briefly with the use of drugs as tools in psychiatric research. Hallucinogens and psychostimulants have no established therapeutic applications in psychiatry and will only be mentioned in connection with their psychotomimetic actions. Alcohol, barbiturates and opiates have important actions on mood and mental processes but are virtually obsolete as psychotherapeutic agents. These drugs are commonly used illicitly, and cause drug dependence, a topic which is dealt with elsewhere in this book. A consideration of the treatment of mental disorders specifically associated with senility and organic brain disease is also outside the scope of this chapter.

General perspective

The drug revolution in psychiatry

Notwithstanding important advances in understanding mental disorders made by Freud, Kraepelin, Bleuler and others, psychiatry in the first half of the twentieth century was dominated by therapeutic nihilism, particularly in dealing with those severe forms of mental disorders known as the functional psychoses. The psychoses involve marked changes in thought and feeling, and diminished contact with reality. Although lacking the pronounced deterioration in cognitive and intellectual capacities characteristic of organic brain dysfunction (delirium and dementia), schizophrenic and other psychotic patients were usually found to be beyond the reach of the new psycho-therapeutic methods of Freud and others, which principally relied on increasing patients' insight into their condition. So by default, pre-dominantly physical methods of treatment were used for dealing with these patients. This was a step backward in the wake of a revolution, since the lessons of earlier pioneers were forgotten. In the 1790s Pinel had espoused the principle and practice of 'moral treatment' for the insane, and apparently demonstrated that humane and personal attention could do much to ameliorate the condition of psychotic patients (Greenblatt, 1978). In contrast to this and other, admittedly exceptional, early enlightened approaches, psychiatrists in the recent past were tackling the problem of the mentally ill by using regimes of harsh physical restraint and containment which were closer to torture than therapy, in institutions more like prisons than hospitals. The widespread use of drugs like bromides, chloral, paraldehyde and barbiturates, which all have relatively non-specific depressant effects on the brain, was justified not because they ameliorated mental dis-order and distress, but largely because patients were more easily managed by overworked and ill-trained attendants. The detrimental effect of these drugs on patients' physical health, and the further impairment of intellectual and social life which they produced, counted for little in environments where physical and social im-poverishment were common, and a poor prognosis was generally accepted as inevitable.

The failure of psychiatrists to offer any effective physical remedies for the mentally ill had produced by the 1930s two paradoxical results. Firstly, it strengthened the belief that all mental illness, including the functional psychoses, could only ultimately be under-stood in psychodynamic terms, even though therapists who put psychoanalytical theories into practice had largely washed their hands of the psychoses. Secondly, it opened the way to even more drastic and ill-conceived means of physical treatment, such as psychosurgery and insulin coma therapy. If such procedures had any benefit at all, it probably resulted from the extra care and personal attention that patients received. However, electro-convulsive therapy (ECT) emerged at this time, and represented the first major advance in the treatment of the psychoses, especially those with a marked affective component. Although today some still maintain that ECT is as unscientific, harmful and ineffective as the discredited physical treatments used in the past, careful evaluation of modern ECT has confirmed its value and relative safety in severe depressive illness, even though the mechanism of its therapeutic effect is poorly understood (Crow and Johnstone, 1979).

This dispiriting state of affairs continued into the 1950s when the start of a remarkable new era coincided with the chance discovery of tricyclic antischizophrenic and antidepressant drugs, and with the introduction of monoamine oxidase inhibitors and lithium salts into psychiatric practice. In many cases, the new drugs enabled symptoms of mental illness to be selectively brought under control without markedly impairing alertness and intellectual functions. Partly as a direct result of the new drugs' effectiveness, and partly no doubt as a result of the spirit of optimism which their use engendered, attempts to improve the physical and social environment in mental hospitals received a new impetus, and patients were helped to learn new work and social skills within the limits of their disabilities. Long-term institutional care was deemed unnecessary for many mental patients, and was being rapidly phased out by the early 1960s. Even though drugs helped rather than cured, patients who would have shown gradual deterioration in hospital were allowed some semblance of normal life outside. However, it was realized from the start that social reforms in managing mental patients were equally if not more important than the direct benefits resulting from the new pharmacotherapy.

Drugs and 'Alternative Psychiatry'

The breakdown of old, entrenched ideas about the nature and management of mental illness also provided the fertilizer for an 'alternative' movement in psychiatry which grew up and flourished in the 1960s. This rejected the notion that disease processes underlie mental disorders. Mental illness, it argued, was a myth, perpetrated by doctors in order to disguise what amounted to a form of protest by the individual faced with intolerable problems of adaptation and conformity to a 'sick' society (Szasz, 1967). Drugs used by conventional psychiatrists were viewed at best as symptomatic remedies for socially unacceptable thoughts, feelings and behaviour, and at worst, as 'chemical strait-jackets'. The implication was that the use of drugs could impede rather than promote recovery from mental disorders. It was argued that rather than suppressing them with drugs, mental symptoms should be used constructively. By working with, and working through mental disorders, psychic conflicts, which were believed to be at their source, could be identified and eliminated.

These ideas represented a sort of rearguard action by psycho-analytically oriented therapists against the medical model of mental illness. Today most of the arguments seem over-inflated, rhetorical, and, particularly with regard to psychotic conditions, frankly misguided. It is now widely accepted that when used appropriately, drugs can be instruments of liberation rather than repression, freeing the patient from the crushing tyranny of disordered thought and feeling. However, the debate was valuable in that it ensured that psychosocial factors relevant to the causes and management of mental disorders were not neglected at a time when an upsurge of new knowledge about physico-chemical brain processes might otherwise have resulted in an over materialistic view. Secondly, it focused attention on many ethical problems surrounding the use of psychotherapeutic drugs, particularly whether drug treatments should be given without patients' consent (Szasz, 1963). Much controversy continues to surround this particular issue (Berger, 1978), but further discussion of it is not possible here.

Biological psychiatry: conceptualizing mental illness and the ways in which drugs can help

Mental illnesses can be defined as syndromes of behavioural and mental phenomena with specific common characteristics which (a) represent deviations from social and cultural norms, (b) place the individual at a biological disadvantage, and (c) involve the experience of distress and suffering. Thoughts, feelings or behaviour may be deviant or undesirable but cannot be 'diseased' in any objective sense. However, the basic premise of the medical model is that the defining features of mental illness are the reflection of brain processes which are maladaptive in that they cause impairment of fundamental biological functions (e.g. social behaviour, sleep, appetite, libido) and that this threatens the individual's survival.

At present, these brain processes are largely hypothetical. Despite extensive research, no pathognomonic lesion in the brain has yet been found to characterize mental disorders such as major affective illness or schizophrenia, and these conditions are still principally diagnosed on the basis of the patients' behaviour and verbalized thoughts and feelings. However, physical changes accompanying mental disorders can be useful supplementary aids to diagnosis, since they often give pointers to prognosis and treatment response. Even in mental disorders where somatic features or progressive deterioration are absent, there are reasons for believing in the existence of underlying physical pathogenic mechanisms. For example, although the manifestations of mental illness are quite variable, characteristic features which cut across marked differences in personality type and cultural background are discernible, and in fact are the mainstay of diagnosis. Secondly, conditions like schizophrenia and major affective illness usually have a family history, due in large extent to the inheritance of genetic factors which increase an individual's susceptibility to the disorder. Thirdly, abnormal mental states resembling the primary functional psychoses sometimes accompany physical diseases which involve the brain, either directly (e.g. in temporal lobe epilepsy, multiple sclerosis and disseminated lupus erythematosis), or indirectly (e.g. in hypo- and hyperthyroidism). Fourthly, a number of drugs such as antihypertensives (reserpine, α-methyl dopa), appetite suppressants (amphetamine, fenfluramine), and corticosteroids, sometimes precipitate severe disturbances of mood, and a state closely resembling paranoid schizophrenia can follow prolonged ingestion of high doses of amphetamine. Fifthly, and most important, the selective reduction of symptoms by psychotherapeutic drugs in many (but not all) cases of mental illness argues strongly for the direct or indirect involvement of physiochemical processes.

A useful conceptual model of mental processes is provided by the computer programme (Figure 7.1), which in effect represents an updating of the old materialist view of the mind–brain relationship. This is in contrast to 'dualist' concepts in which mind and brain are believed to exist quite independently. Programme malfunctions analogous to features of mental illness may arise because 'faulty' instructions have been fed into the computer, or because a failure occurs in one of the computer's circuits. In addition, one type of fault may lead to the other. The model stresses that the neurotic–psychotic distinction used in diagnosis (actually a reflection of illness severity) may be related, but is not identical to the psychogenic–neurogenic aetiological dimension. The analogy also helps in conceptualizing the role of drugs and other physical treatments in the management of

Computer analogy	Clinical classification	Treatment model	Practical implications
Software malfunction only	Reactive/psychogenic functional disorder	Alter input conditions, and/or reprogramme, with or without partial circuit 'shut-down'	Await spontaneous recovery; alter life circumstances; increase insight; remove psychic conflicts; identify and modify maladaptive behaviour. Use drugs to induce mental states conducive to psychotherapy or behaviour modification
Software malfunction and secondary hardware defect	Reactive/psychogenic with neurogenic features	Treat as above to allow eventual self-correction of hardware defect, and/or intervene more directly to repair defect	If possible use drugs with selective effects on specific mental dysfunctions arising out of putative pathognomonic lesions in brain structure or function; drugs with non-selective effects on mental dysfunctions may help patient rehabilitation by suppressing disruptive or unacceptable behaviour arising from unremediable residual or progressive mental illness
Primary hardware defect and secondary programme faults	Neurogenic (endogenous) features predominate (covert organic brain dysfunction)	Repair hardware defect, if possible, and reprogramme; otherwise isolate malfunctioning circuits, and reprogramme for less demanding tasks	

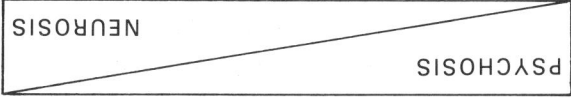

NEUROSIS

PSYCHOSIS

Fig. 7.1 Computer programme faults can provide analogies for mental disorders and their management, including the use of psychotherapeutic drugs.

mental disturbances. However attractive the idea, it seems unlikely that psychotherapeutic drugs correct or repair specific, but as yet unidentified, brain lesions which are directly responsible for mental disorders. More likely, drugs act on brain processes which, in concert with other factors (some intrinsic to brain function, and others extrinsic, e.g. environmentally determined), lead indirectly to amelioration of mental disturbance. One important implication is that following drug action on relevant brain processes, improvement in mental state may not be immediate or inevitable, but will depend on demolishing (reprogramming) the mental and behavioural super-structures which have developed around the basic biological defect. In other words, psychotherapeutic drugs may help create or restore the physiochemical conditions in the brain which are necessary before a return to a normal mental state can begin, just as acute cerebral ischaemia after a stroke must be relieved, or allowed to subside, before undamaged brain tissue can be 're-educated' to take over part of the function of brain cells irreparably lost. The actual remission of mental symptoms may rely on environmental and social circumstances affecting psychological and neurobiological processes in the same way that controlled exercises and rehabilitation programmes are necessary in order to optimize recovery of function in the stroke patient. An additional complication is that the drug effects which set the stage for mental recovery may also be indirect and take time to develop fully.

Psychotherapeutic drugs in current use

Classification

As described in Chapter 1, psychotherapeutic drugs can be broadly classified according to their principal usage into antianxiety, anti-depressant and antipsychotic (neuroleptic) agents. Within the major groups, there are a number of subclasses based on shared chemical structure and/or pharmacological properties. There are differences between and within subclasses with respect to therapeutic potency and the ability to induce certain side-effects, both adverse and advantageous, depending on the circumstances. In most cases, these clinical differences can be related to the chemical and pharma-cological properties used to classify the drugs. However, it is much less certain whether these properties can be related, directly or indirectly, to the drugs' principal therapeutic actions on 'core' features of the disorders they are used to treat. Although it is a rather sweeping generalization, there are no striking differences in therapeutic efficacy within the three major drug groups when potency and pharmacokinetic considerations, and the preferential response of some patients to particular drugs, are taken into account. Possible exceptions to this generalization are the benzodiazepines in the anxiolytic group, and lithium in the antidepressant group.

Antianxiety drugs

A large number of centrally active drugs produce sedation, the term formerly used to imply a reduction in anxiety. In most cases, undesirable drowsiness and psychomotor impairment occur as well. The benzodiazepines, which are by far the most widely used antianxiety drugs, are often effective at doses which do not cause drowsiness. The term 'tranquillizer' is commonly used for drugs with this characteristic. However, the difference between the benzodiazepines and the older barbiturate type of anxiolytic in this respect is probably overrated. Benzodiazepines are preferred by anxious patients, apparently because they restore a more normal mood state, even in the presence of drowsiness (Lader, 1979). The most striking advantage of the benzodiazepines over other sedative drugs is their greater safety. A fairly light state of unconsciousness, with anterograde amnesia on recovery, is all that can be produced even with high doses of these drugs. By contrast, profound and frequently fatal cerebral, respiratory, and cardiovascular depression occur after quite small overdoses of barbiturates.

Self-assertiveness may be increased by benzodiazepine in people who are otherwise timid and inhibited, but there is nothing comparable with the release of aggression that is often produced by alcohol. Similarly, the euphoric sensations associated with low, disinhibiting doses of alcohol and barbiturates are almost entirely absent, which partly explains why benzodiazepines are less likely to be deliberately abused. However psychological dependence on their anxiolytic action can occur, and tolerance and physical dependence have been demonstrated when benzodiazepines are given in high doses over long periods. When the drugs are stopped, their effects are slow to wear off, so that withdrawal symptoms, if they occur, are delayed and relatively mild. However it is sometimes difficult to distinguish between the benzodiazepine abstinence syndrome and a recrudescence of anxiety.

Some benzodiazepines are also useful anticonvulsants, and all cause a reduction in muscle tone due to an action on the spinal cord. A reduction in muscle spasm associated with anxiety may contribute indirectly to the beneficial effect of the drugs on mood.

The antianxiety properties of benzodiazepines are frequently and effectively exploited for treating insomnia, since anxiety is a common reason for difficulty in falling asleep. For this application, any drug-induced drowsiness is a positive advantage. The normal pattern of sleep is less markedly disturbed by the benzodiazepines than it is by other hypnotic drugs. However hangover effects still occur, probably because many benzodiazepines have active metabolites with long half-lives (typically 50 hours or more). Although it would seem logical to prescribe short-acting drugs for use as hypnotics, long-acting drugs like nitrazepam are still promoted and frequently prescribed for this purpose (Table 7.1). There appear to be no important qualitative differences between any of the benzodiazepines available, at least with respect to their tranquillizing and hypnotic effects. Many drugs even share the same active metabolites (desmethyldiazepam and oxazepam). With repeated administration, the effects of the metabolites tend to predominate over those of the parent drugs, reducing any differences between drugs still further.

Anxiety and agitation may be prominent features of depressive illness, in which case they usually respond to treatment with anti-depressant drugs. Some antidepressants cause drowsiness, particularly early on in treatment, and this may be an advantage in depressed patients who are agitated. It is possible that certain anti-depressant drugs have antianxiety effects independent of their main action. Thus phobic anxiety and panic attacks, disorders which are usually distinct from depressive illness, are helped by monoamine oxidase inhibitors and by tricyclic antidepressants, especially imipramine and clomipramine. Neuroleptic 'major tranquillizers' in low doses are also sometimes used for treating anxiety, their chief advantage being the avoidance of drug dependence. However, the risk of neurotoxic and other serious adverse effects occurring with long-term treatment, even at low doses, usually discourages their use.

Many of the bodily sensations caused by, and often contributing to, anxiety are mediated by β-adrenergic pathways. These somatic complaints can be reduced by β-adrenoceptor blocking drugs, which may

Table 7.1   Short and long-acting benzodiazepines

Short-acting	Long-acting
Triazolam*	Chlordiazepoxide
	Diazepam
Lorazepam†	Clorazepate
Oxazepam†	Medazepam
Temazepam†*	Ketazolam
	Flurazepam*
	Clonazepam
	Clobazam
	Nitrazepam†*

*   Promoted as hypnotics
†   Drugs with inactive metabolites

be very helpful in selected cases (Lader, 1979). Propranolol and some other β-blockers used in treating anxiety enter the brain and cause drowsiness and disturbed sleep. These central effects may involve blockade of serotonin receptors as well as β-adrenoceptors, but it is not clear how they modify or contribute to the drugs' anxiolytic potential.

Antidepressant drugs

The majority of clinically important antidepressants are monoamine reuptake inhibitors (MARI). The original members of this group (e.g. imipramine, amitriptyline) have a tricyclic chemical structure, and a wide spectrum of pharmacological properties, similar to those of the phenothiazine neuroleptics. Newer additions are chemically and pharmacologically dissimilar in various degrees. None of these differences have resulted in any important improvements in anti-depressant efficacy. About 60 to 80% of depressed patients benefit from treatment with MARI drugs, typically after a delay of several weeks. A feature of the drugs is their long action, so that a single dose at night usually suffices. Side-effects are numerous and include postural hypotension and sedation, probably related to blockade of peripheral and central α-adrenoceptors respectively, and autonomic symptoms typical of cholinergic blockade (e.g. dry mouth, blurred vision, constipation, and urinary retention). Dysrhythmias and other cardiotoxic effects may be a problem, particularly in patients with pre-existing heart disease, and are probably related to the drugs' indirect sympathomimetic action in the heart. Newer drugs appear to retain the effectiveness of the originals, but with fewer side-effects (Table 7.2).

Most MARI drugs predominantly affect the reuptake of noradrenaline into peripheral and central nerve endings. Some drugs which are weak in this respect have active metabolites which are more potent. Other drugs increase synaptic levels of noradrenaline by additional mechanisms (e.g. mianserin blocks presynaptic α-2 adrenoceptors which inhibit noradrenaline release). Clomipramine and zimelidine are the only drugs which have a marked effect on the neuronal re-uptake of serotonin. Patients in whom there is biochemical evidence of reduced serotonin turnover in the brain may respond better to MARI and other drugs which increase synaptic levels of serotonin as well as those of noradrenaline. Patients with normal serotonin turnover, who may be clinically indistinguishable, seem to respond best to drugs with a more selective effect on noradrenaline (Goodwin et al., 1978). With the exception of nomifensine, all MARI drugs are ineffective as inhibitors of dopamine reuptake. This special property of nomifensine probably explains its psychostimulant properties, whereas most MARI drugs are sedative. However, antidepressant drugs may produce an increase in dopaminergic transmission by promoting the gradual de-sensitization of inhibitory receptors on presynaptic neurones (Chiodo and Antelman, 1980).

Other antidepressant drugs are probably less effective clinically than the MARI drugs, and in addition have a number of other dis-advantages. For example, monoamine oxidase inhibitors (MAOI) may lead to serious adverse reactions with certain other drugs, or after ingestion of food containing tyramine (e.g. cheese). However they may be useful when other antidepressant drugs have failed, and are possibly the treatment of choice in hypochondriacal or hysterical depressive conditions. Indoleamine precursors such as L-tryptophan and 5-hydroxytryptophan have been proposed as antidepressants, but have doubtful efficacy. Although they are safe, they are unpleasant to take because of gastro-intestinal side-effects. Combining these pre-cursors with MAOI or MARI drugs may cause a more selective increase in serotonin availability in the brain, and an enhanced therapeutic effect in certain patients.

Table 7.2 Clinical properties of some antidepressant drugs compared with imipramine

Antidepressant drug	Speed of action	Anxiolytic effect	Sedative effect	Anticholinergic effect	Cardiotoxicity	Epileptogenic effect
Amitriptyline	same	better	more	same	same	same
Maprotiline	faster(?)	same	more	same/less	less	greater
Protriptyline	faster(?)	same	same	more	less	same
Trazodone	same	better	more	less	less	same
Mianserin	same	better(?)	more	less	less	same
Nomifensine	same	better(?)	less	less	less	less(?)
Viloxazine	faster(?)	same(?)	less(?)	less(?)*	less	greater(?)
Zimelidine†	same	better(?)	less	less*	less	same

* Causes nausea

† No longer availabe in UK

Antidepressant medication is usually continued at full dosage for several months after symptoms have subsided, and is then gradually withdrawn. If there is a history of frequent or prolonged previous episodes of depression, long-term maintenance therapy with MARI drugs may be effective in reducing subsequent attacks. However, where there is a history of mania or hypomania as well as depression (bipolar illness), lithium may be a more suitable alternative for prophylaxis. MARI antidepressants have little protective value against mania, and may even provoke it in susceptible individuals. By contrast lithium, as well as reducing recurrent depression (unipolar illness), is even more effective against both manic and depressive episodes in bipolar illness (Coppen and Peet, 1979).

Mania is a condition in which the retardation of thought and motor activity typical of depression is reversed. Although mood is usually heightened, features of depressive illness such as hostility and delusional guilt are just below the surface. It is likely that mania, and depression with a history of mania, are both manifestations of the same fundamental disorder (bipolar affective illness). Depression without mania (unipolar illness) may either be a separate entity, or, as now seems more likely, a less severe form of bipolar illness (Sachar and Baron, 1979).

Lithium is the treatment of choice in mania, having a highly selective normalizing action in the 70 to 80 per cent of patients who respond. However, its action is slow, taking up to ten days to have full effect, and a more rapid response can be obtained by adding a neuroleptic drug such as haloperidol. Although very speedy and effective in reducing manic hyperactivity, neuroleptics are somewhat less selective than lithium, since sedation may be produced without complete control of manic symptoms (Shopsin et al., 1979). Lithium may also be effective in dealing with depressive episodes in some bipolar patients (Paykel, 1979). Lithium produces numerous side-effects, e.g. on the kidney, thyroid gland, bone marrow and nervous system, and toxicity is easily produced if plasma levels become too high (Coppen and Peet, 1979). However, higher plasma levels may be tolerated by acutely manic patients, and lower levels may be needed to avoid toxicity in patients on lithium prophylaxis. The diverse side-effects of lithium are not surprising in view of the many biological systems (particularly those associated with cell membranes) affected by this simple inorganic ion, which has properties in common with sodium, potassium, calcium, and magnesium. By contrast, the highly selective and unique spectrum of psychotherapeutic actions shown by lithium is both a puzzle and a powerful challenge for psychobiological research.

Antipsychotic drugs

These drugs have the unique ability to improve psychotic states, the central feature of which is a distorted perception of reality. The prototype of this group of drugs is chlorpromazine, a 'tricyclic' phenothiazine compound which was discovered around 1950 during the search for sedative antihistamine drugs. Chlorpromazine was found to have a very large range of pharmacological actions and clinical uses (hence its trade name, 'Largactil'), including anti-adrenergic, antiemetic, antioedematous, and antipyretic properties, and potentiation of analgesic and central depressant drugs. However, the most striking actions of chlorpromazine were observed in psychiatric patients, and first described in 1952 by Delay and Deniker, who used the term 'neuroleptic' for drugs with the following properties. Firstly, a 'major tranquillizing' action which involves the blunting of motor and emotional reactions to the environment, including a reduction in anxiety and agitation, but without marked drowsiness or intellectual impairment. Secondly, the ability to produce a number of neurological disorders of movement (extra-pyramidal effects), some of which resemble those seen in Parkinson's disease, e.g. resting tremor, limb rigidity, shuffling gait, etc., whereas others have a more unusual character, e.g. acute spasms of the muscles in the tongue, face, neck, etc., and a subjective sense of restlessness leading to compulsive fidgeting. Thirdly, a selective, albeit delayed, reduction in psychotic symptoms and associated behaviour. 'Positive' psychotic features such as hallucinations, delusions, disorganized thinking, hostility and motor hyperactivity show the most striking therapeutic response, but social withdrawal, apathy, and even catatonic states usually improve as well, despite the sedative and cataleptic properties of neuroleptic drugs.

Adverse effects of chlorpromazine and related drugs are numerous and include postural hypotension and other antiadrenergic and anticholinergic autonomic effects, weight gain, hormonal disturbances, photosensitivity and skin pigmentation, eczema, cardiotoxicity, convulsions, jaundice and, rarely, agranulocytosis. Most obvious however are the sedation and movement disorders which are an integral part of neuroleptic action as first defined by Delay and Deniker. However, it was soon realized that these effects may be dissociated from an antipsychotic action, because tolerance to the sedative and parkinsonian effects of chlorpromazine occurs as treatment is prolonged, whereas the antipsychotic action tends to build up. More striking dissociations between neuroleptic effects are seen with some more recently discovered potent antipsychotic drugs which have only slight sedative-anxiolytic actions, but marked parkinsonian effects. Also there are even newer drugs which are effective, albeit rather weak, antipsychotic agents despite the virtual absence of other neuroleptic characteristics (Table 7.3).

The ideal antipsychotic drug has yet to be discovered. Meanwhile existing neuroleptic drugs are useful stopgaps, since their extrapyramidal effects can be managed in various ways. Firstly, as already mentioned, most neuroleptic-induced movement disorders tend to wane over time. However, this is not usually sufficient in practice, because there is often a somewhat paradoxical increase in extrapyramidal effects when the dose of neuroleptic is reduced from the high levels used for initial management of psychoses to the more moderate ones used for continuation therapy (Hollister, 1978). One practical solution to the problem is to use additional drugs with central anticholinergic effects which partially cancel neuroleptic actions on the extrapyramidal system of the brain (basal ganglia). However, there is some evidence that anticholinergic drugs also slightly reduce the antipsychotic component of neuroleptic action. An alternative is to use lower doses of neuroleptic drugs which retain a sufficient antipsychotic action without troublesome extrapyramidal effects. Some neuroleptics (e.g. thioridizine) have marked anticholinergic properties in their own right, which probably explains the lower incidence of extrapyramidal effects associated with their use. Clozapine, an antipsychotic drug not generally available because of its toxic effects on bone marrow, produces few if any extrapyramidal effects. Although it exhibits anticholinergic properties *in vitro*, this does not seem to be the case *in vivo*. Like an even more specific antipsychotic drug called sulpiride, clozapine is a very weak neuroleptic. However, both drugs probably have other properties which selectively boost the limbic but not the extrapyramidal component of their actions, so accounting for their selective antipsychotic effects.

About a quarter of patients with schizophrenia recover completely, whereas another quarter remain affected for the rest of their lives,

Table 7.3 Clinical properties of different classes of antipsychotic drugs

Class of drug	Typical daily dose (mg/day)	NEUROLEPTIC ACTIONS			Anti-cholinergic effects	Postural hypotension
		Anti-psychotic*	Sedative-anxiolytic	Extra-pyramidal		
PHENOTHIAZINES						
with aliphatic side-chain						
e.g. chlorpromazine	500	+ + +	+ + +	+ +	+ +	+ +
with piperidine side-chain						
e.g. thioridizine	400	+ + +	+ + +	+	+ + +	+ + +
with piperazine side-chain						
e.g. fluphenazine‡	20	+ + +	+	+ + +	+	+
BUTYROPHENONES						
e.g. haloperidol†	20	+ + +	+	+ + +	+	+
DIPHENYLBUTYLPIPERIDINES						
e.g. pimozide	10	+ + +	+ / 0	+	+ / 0	+ / 0
BENZAMIDES						
e.g. sulpiride	1000	+ + +	0	+	+ (?)	+ / 0 (?)
DIBENZODIAZEPINES						
e.g. clozapine§	200	+ + +	+ + +	0	+ + (?)	+ + +

* All drugs adjusted to equivalent therapeutic doses
‡ Depot form available for maintenance therapy
† Now available in depot form
§ Not generally available in UK

and are only marginally helped by drugs. Even in the remainder of patients who have an intermediate prognosis, without treatment the relapse rate can be as high as 80 per cent in the year following recovery from an acute episode of schizophrenia. However maintenance treatment with neuroleptics may reduce this figure by more than half (Leff and Wing, 1971). Apart from the adverse effects already mentioned, long-term neuroleptic use brings the risk of a potentially irreversible neurotoxic condition called tardive dyskinesia. This condition involves involuntary tic-like movements mostly of the face, mouth and tongue, and occurs in about 20 per cent of chronic schizophrenics. Unlike the extrapyramidal effects of neuroleptics, tardive dyskinesia is not helped in the short term by reducing neuroleptic dose, nor by giving anticholinergic drugs. In fact, in both cases tardive dyskinesia may get worse. The observation that tardive dyskinesia may occur in schizophrenics who have never received neuroleptic drugs suggests that the condition may be a neurological complication of chronic schizophrenia, which is aggravated rather than caued by neuroleptic drugs.

Probably over half the patients put on long-term drug therapy do not take their drugs as prescribed, if at all. In view of this, the introduction of long-acting preparations of neuroleptic drugs has greatly helped the management of chronic schizophrenia. The drugs are given as slow release intramuscular injections, with a duration of action of up to four weeks. Extrapyramidal effects may still be a problem, and will require daily pill taking, since it is not feasible to use a depot anticholinergic drug.

Uses and abuses of psychotherapeutic drugs

Are drugs overused?

Assessing the risks and benefits of psychotherapeutic drugs presents formidable difficulties. All currently available psychotherapeutic drugs can produce serious adverse effects, some potentially fatal (e.g. convulsions and cardiotoxicity with tricyclic drugs). Particular doubts about the value of long-term psychotherapeutic drug use centre upon the failure of most drugs (lithium may be an exception) to alter fundamentally the course of chronic mental disorders, combined with an increased risk of serious adverse effects. In view of this, over-reliance on drugs, especially in the case of relatively trivial and self-limiting mental problems, is both unnecessary and undesirable. Persistent and troublesome deviations from 'mental health' are often encountered in general medical practice, but in many instances there is no clear evidence of 'disease' except in a literal sense. It is arguable that non-medical approaches to management are more appropriate in these cases. However, people with intractable problems continue to come to doctors for help, and it is usually out of expediency that doctors resort to drug treatment.

As many as one in five doctors' prescriptions are for psycho-therapeutic drugs, mostly of the anti-anxiety or sedative type (Baldessarini, 1980). Probably about 15 per cent of the general population take an anxiolytic sedative drug for 'nerves' or 'depression' at least once during a year, and nearly two-thirds of these people take drugs regularly (Silverstone and Turner, 1982). It may be that the troubles of the modern world make us particularly anxious and despondent, but the belief, largely fostered by doctors in the past, that there is a pill for every problem has also probably contributed to the high demand for psychotherapeutic drugs. Of course unpleasant and in-capacitating mood states warrant attention, and in some cases require treatment with drugs, but in a consumer society, psychotherapeutic drugs are often regarded merely as products of modern technology, promoted and sold to make life easier. Not surprisingly, many take it for granted that efficacy and safety are guaranteed.

Are drugs effective?

There are considerable difficulties in evaluating the effectiveness of psychotherapeutic drugs in controlled 'double-blind' clinical trials. Once a drug is believed to have some efficacy, assessment of exactly how much may be problematical, because this necessitates a comparison with a placebo. Withholding active treatment may be regarded as unethical, so, as a compromise, comparison is often made with another, better established drug. Changes in subjective complaints are difficult to measure reliably, particularly as they tend to show marked fluctuations in both the short and longer term. In acute conditions, the spontaneous recovery rate can be high, so drug efficacy may be overestimated if adequate controls are not used. On the other hand, there is considerable between-subject variation in the amount and duration of drug treatment needed to produce an optimum therapeutic response. Unless a flexible design is adopted, clinical trials may reject potentially useful drugs as 'no better than placebos', especially if the numbers of patients in the samples are small, or if, as is usual, it is doubtful that all patients are taking the treatment as prescribed. A common mistake is to assume that failure to find a statistically significant difference in efficacy is adequate proof that drug and placebo are equal (Hollister, 1978).

A further complication in drug assessment is the possible heterogeneity of mental disorders in patients grouped together for clinical trials: it seems that broad similarities at a clinical level may obscure important biological differences between patients. This may account for some of the striking variations in response to drug treatment which are sometimes seen. Psychotherapeutic drugs for which efficacy in some patients is well established may still be ineffective in a quarter or more of all patients considered eligible for treatment. Apparent inconsistency of drug action may be misinterpreted as no useful action at all. However, there is a danger of arguing in circles, because a differential response to drugs is one of the main pillars supporting the idea of biological heterogeneity within the major diagnostic groups of mental illness. The identification of independent clinical, epidemiological and neurobiological criteria which correlate with differential response to drug treatments is an important area of contemporary psychiatric research (Goodwin *et al.*, 1978; Murphy *et al.*, 1978).

Sometimes individual patients who failed to benefit from a particular drug will respond to another drug, which, as far as can be ascertained, is very similar with respect to its clinical effects and spectrum of pharmacological actions. A possible explanation for this type of observation is that the drugs in question differ with respect to an as yet undiscovered action which is crucial for a therapeutic effect in the patient concerned. However, this rather seems to overstretch the concept of biological heterogeneity existing within a given class of mental disorders. A more likely explanation is that the pharmacokinetic and metabolic fate of closely related drugs may differ, and such differences are accentuated in some patients. By implication, only drugs which reach an adequate level in the relevant tissues of a particular patient, or result in the formation of a certain metabolite, will produce a therapeutic response. If a drug fails to produce the required response, substitution rather than addition of another drug is the best principle. Concurrent administration of two or more drugs from the same class is rarely if ever justified.

When are drugs indicated?

As a general rule, the clearest indication for psychotherapeutic drugs is in the treatment of specific psychiatric conditions such as schizophrenia, mania, depression ('melancholia') and pathological anxiety, in which the patients' symptoms lead more or less directly to suffering and disability. The indiscriminate use of powerful drugs in situations where their value for the patient is not reasonably well established is to be deplored. Schizophrenic and depressed patients typically feel more normal once appropriate, specific drug therapy has been established, whereas people without these particular disorders usually feel unpleasantly abnormal and impaired when given the same drugs. Similarly, sufferers from incapacitating anxiety often cope and feel better on drug therapy which in normal people causes intolerable drowsiness. An extreme form of misuse of psychotherapeutic drugs which is sanctioned by some totalitarian states is the forcible administration of large doses of sedative tranquillizers to political prisoners.

Short-term versus long-term treatment

Mental disorders with an acute onset are often associated with dramatic symptoms, but typically get better on their own in a high percentage of cases. Drugs may speed recovery, but the advantage of this for the patient may be outweighed by the risk of serious adverse effects. However, mental illness is usually highly distressing for all concerned, and so prompt relief is a priority.

In schizophrenia and depressive illness, a relapsing course with spontaneous remissions is common. Drugs which facilitate remission can also be used successfully as maintenance therapy, so reducing the frequency and severity of relapse in a proportion of patients. The most striking example is the use of the antimanic agent lithium to prevent recurrences of both mania and depression (Coppen and Peet, 1979). In any individual the chances of relapse without drug treatment cannot be known for certain, but they can be gauged with reasonable accuracy from the results of epidemiological research which relates prognosis to features of the presenting illness and the patient's environment. In patients who are thought unlikely to relapse, long-term drug therapy is obviously best avoided. For the rest, the protective value of maintenance therapy may be very different depending on the type of illness and other circumstances.

For example, schizophrenics who are particularly likely to relapse if subjected to an unremediably intense emotional atmosphere at home, may benefit considerably from maintenance therapy with anti-psychotic drugs, despite the attendant risk of adverse drug reactions (e.g. tardive dyskinesia). In other types of schizophrenia ('type II'), there seems to be an inexorable deterioration in the patients' mental state, which becomes dominated by 'negative' features such as emotional flattening and social withdrawal. Neurological abnormali-ties including movement disorders and cerebral atrophy may be present, and not surprisingly, there may be cognitive and intellectual impairment as well. This deterioration does not seem to be caused by drugs or other physical treatments, but neither is it significantly helped by them (Owens and Johnstone, 1980).

Non-psychotic conditions such as pathological anxiety and obses-sive−compulsive neurosis can also run a chronic, although not neces-sarily deteriorating, course. Usually these conditions seem to arise out of fundamental and more or less permanent features of the person-ality, and the value of long-term drug therapy is limited. Drugs are most useful for dealing with acute exacerbations which are often precipitated by transient life crises. Where excessive anxiety is episodic, or associated with specific circumstances, it is usually better to use anxiolytic drugs when most needed, rather than to give them continuously, when tolerance and dependence may become a prob-lem.

Choosing the right drug

The decision of which type of psychotherapeutic drug to use in any particular case is made on the basis of the patient's overall diagnosis. This may seem obvious, but there is a temptation to use the same drugs in conditions which, although fundamentally different, some-times have symptoms in common. For example, the most appropriate treatment for a patient with delusions and hallucinations may be an antidepressant rather than an antipsychotic if the overall clinical picture suggests a predominantly affective disorder. However, both types of drug may be used together when psychotic and affective features coexist. Although some antipsychotic drugs may exacerbate or provoke depressive symptoms, others (e.g. flupenthixol) have anti-depressant properties in their own right. Most antipsychotic drugs are very effective in the management of mania and other excited delusional states, and this can only partly be explained by the sedative properties which some possess. In other words, the beneficial effects of these drugs are not restricted to schizophrenic psychoses. By contrast, the antimanic action of lithium appears to be both selective and specific in that lithium can restore the mood of manic patients to near normal, and yet has little or no value in schizophrenia (Shopsin *et al.*, 1979).

Antidepressant drugs frequently benefit patients who appear predominantly anxious (Johnstone *et al.*, 1980), possibly because most pathological anxiety and psychogenic depression are manifestations of the same basic disorder. However, depression does not usually respond to anxiolytic drugs even when agitation and anxiety are prominent features. Occasionally, anxiety is an early presenting feature of schizophrenia or organic brain dysfunction, and in these cases treatment should be directed at the underlying condition.

Increased awareness that drug-responsive depressive illness underlies many mental and psychosomatic complaints has caused a general increase in the use of antidepressant drugs. Some of these drugs are quite toxic, particularly in overdose. Since depressive illnesses are usually self-limiting disorders, it could be argued that dangerous drug treatments are not justified. However, antidepressant drugs can usually speed the rate of recovery considerably, especially if environmental circumstances are less than ideal. As suicide is an ever-present risk in depressive illness, appropriate use of antidepressant drugs may be life saving, so long as precautions are taken against patients deliberately overdosing with the drugs. Endogenous (neurogenic) depression, which has pronounced somatic features such as weight loss, early morning wakening and endocrine dysfunctions, is often said to respond better than other types of depressive disorder to drug treatment. However, this difference is not always found in controlled trials (Murphy *et al.*, 1978). Depression *without* marked somatic features undoubtedly does often benefit from treatment with antidepressant drugs (Paykel, 1979). Psychotic symptoms (e.g. delusions) are uncommon in these cases, and a psychogenic aetiology is often suggested by stressful life events preceding the illness. Accordingly psychosocial considerations must also feature in patient management.

The use of drugs in psychiatric research

The aim of much psychiatric research is to find new and better drugs and to gain new insights into the nature of the conditions they are used to treat. Advances in knowledge might be expected to precede, and be necessary for, progress in drug therapy, but in fact all effective drugs to date have been discovered by chance, and developed more or less empirically. If a drug is found by serendipity to exert worthwhile and specific therapeutic effects in mental disorders, it is likely to provide a valuable reference point in the search for new treatments and new knowledge. The drug's spectrum of pharmacological actions can be studied in the hope of discovering biological effects, or combinations of effects, which may be linked with its psychotherapeutic properties. If the reference drug is one of several having similar or identical clinical effects, then relevant biological actions should be restricted to these drugs, and be common to all of them. If the members of the reference psychotherapeutic drug group show variations in clinical potency, then corresponding variations in potency should occur in the biological test system which is the presumed target of their specific action. However, allowance may have to be made for differing drug bioavailability in the therapeutic and test situations. Psychotherapeutic actions of drugs are usually delayed, and it is often assumed that chronic rather than acute drug effects are likely to be more relevant for developing theories of the drugs' mechanism of action. This may be true in some cases, but it should not be overemphasized because, as mentioned in an earlier section, the delay before improvement in mental symptoms occurs may be dependent as much or more on psychodynamic factors as on pharmacodynamic ones.

Once specific biological effects of reference psychotherapeutic agents on target systems have been identified, they may be integrated into, or form the basis of, working hypotheses of the biological mechanisms involved in their clinical effects. Formulating testable predictions about how established drugs work is a necessary first step if new and better drugs are to be developed logically rather than by chance. Obviously it helps if there are other grounds for supposing that the identified specific effects of reference drugs are indeed relevant to the biology of mental illness. In many instances this supporting evidence also comes from pharmacological studies. For example, hormonal and autonomic responses to drugs with specific actions on central or peripheral neurotransmitter receptors have suggested that altered sensitivity in some neuronal systems may play a part in the pathogenesis of mental disorders, and may represent the target for psychotherapeutic drug action. Another body of evidence which has been very influential in shaping current ideas about the biology of mental illness centres on the ability of certain drugs with known effects on brain functions to modify or induce mental disorders in humans, or to produce possibly analogous states in animals. Reserpine and amphetamine are two drugs which have been particularly useful in this context, but there are many more examples.

Of course animals cannot communicate their thoughts and feelings directly, but by inference from their behaviour, it does not seem likely that they experience anything closely resembling human mental illness under either natural or experimental conditions. Although mental illness may depend on disruption of brain 'programmes' which are peculiar to humans, it is conceivable that the putative disturbances in brain 'machinery' which underlie some psychiatric disorders can be reproduced in animals, and shown to have specific sensitivity to reference psychotherapeutic drugs. Artificial alterations in brain functions intended to provide animal models of mental illness can either be achieved relatively directly by the use of drugs, neural lesions or electrical and chemical stimulation of the brain, or, more indirectly by manipulation of animals' physical and social environments. Animal tests used to screen new drugs for potential psychotherapeutic properties often rely on these strategies, and are usually validated by their ability to yield few or no false positive or false negative results when using drugs with known psychotherapeutic properties.

There are numerous pitfalls in drug-oriented psychiatric research. Screening tests for psychotherapeutic agents have tended to select new drugs with properties very similar to those of the prototype drugs. The resulting association between certain pharmacological actions and clinical efficacy has understandably been interpreted as cause and effect. However, deliberately engineered variations of these properties have been achieved by chemists and pharmacologists, but sometimes with no obvious changes in psychotherapeutic efficacy. The chance discovery of novel drugs which are as effective as the old has often forced drastic reappraisals of how the drugs exert their clinical effects. The essentially uniform effects of the drugs within each major class of psychotherapeutic agents have fostered the notion of common biological mechanisms of action. Recent basic research with antipsychotic and antidepressant drugs tends to reinforce this idea, although the means by which a final common action is brought about may vary. However, it is possible that drugs yet to be discovered may work quite differently from existing ones, because it is highly unlikely that the brain functions affected by psychotherapeutic drugs are directly, solely, or invariably responsible for recovery from mental illness. It may be that drugs act at various links in the chain of events between physico-chemical processes and specific mental disorders. Even if the mechanisms of action of a given class of psychotherapeutic agents are correctly identified, the question of what physico-chemical processes, if any, are involved in the pathogenesis of the relevant mental disorder is not automatically solved, because those processes may occur at a different link in the chain from the one acted on by the drugs.

References

(References marked * are recommended for general reading.)

Baldessarini, R. J. (1980)* Drugs and the treatment of psychiatric disorders. In A. G. Gilman, L. S. Goodman and A. Gilman (eds) *The Pharmacological Basis of Therapeutics* (6th edn). New York: Macmillan, pp. 391−447.

Berger, P. A. (1978)* Medical treatment of mental illness. *Science 200*: 974−81.

Chiodo, L. A. and Antelman, S. M. (1980) Repeated tricyclics induce a progressive dopamine autoreceptor subsensitivity independent of daily drug treatment. *Nature 287*: 451−4.

Coppen, A. and Peet, M. (1979) The long-term management of patients with affective disorders. In E. S. Paykel and A. Coppen (eds) *Psychopharmacology of Affective Disorders*. Oxford: Oxford Medical Publications, pp. 248−55.

Crow, T. J. and Johnstone, E. C. (1979) Electroconvulsive therapy: efficacy, mechanism of action, and adverse effects. In E. S. Paykel and A. Coppen (eds) *Psychopharmacology of Affective Disorders*. Oxford: Oxford Medical Publications, pp. 108−22.

Goodwin, F. K., Cowdry, R. W. and Webster, M. H. (1978) Predictors of drug response in the affective disorders: towards an integrated approach. In M. A. Lipton, A. DiMascio and K. F. Killam (eds) *Psychopharmacology: A Generation of Progress*. New York: Raven Press, pp. 1277−88.

Greenblatt, M. (1978) Drugs, schizophrenia, and the third revolution. In M. A. Lipton, A. DiMascio and K. F. Killam (eds) *Psychopharmacology: A Generation of Progress*. New York: Raven Press, pp. 1375−80.

Hollister, L. E. (1978)* *Clinical Pharmacology of Psychotherapeutic Drugs*. New York: Churchill Livingstone.

Johnstone, E. C., Owens, D. G. C., Frith, C. D., McPherson, K., Dowie, C., Riley, G. and Gold, A. (1980) Neurotic illness and its response to anxiolytic and antidepressant treatment. *Psychological Medicine 10*: 321−8.

Lader, M. (1979) Anxiety reduction and sedation: psychological theory. *British Journal of Clinical Pharmacology* 7: 99S–105S.

Leff, J. P. and Wing, J. K. (1971) Trial of maintenance therapy in schizophrenia. *British Medical Journal III*: 559–604.

Lipton, M. A., DiMascio, A., and Killam, K. F. (eds) (1978)* *Psychopharmacology: A Generation of Progress*. New York: Raven Press.

Murphy, D. L., Shiling, D. J., and Murray, R. M. (1978) Psychoactive drug responder subgroups: possible contributions to psychiatric classification. In M. A. Lipton, A. DiMascio and K. F. Killam (eds) *Psychopharmacology: A Generation of Progress*. New York: Raven Press, pp. 807–20.

Owens, D. G. C. and Johnstone, E. C. (1980) The disabilities of chronic schizophrenia: their nature and factors contributing to their development. *British Journal of Psychiatry 136*: 384–95.

Paykel, E. S. (1979) Predictors of treatment response. In E. S. Paykel and A. Coppen (eds) *Psychopharmacology of Affective Disorders*. Oxford: Oxford Medical Publications, pp. 193–220.

Paykel, E. S. and Coppen, A. (eds) (1979)* *Psychopharmacology of Affective Disorders*. Oxford: Oxford Medical Publications.

Sachar, E. J. and Baron, M. (1979)* The biology of affective disorders. *Annual Review of Neuroscience 2*: 505–18.

Shopsin, B., Georgotas, A. and Kane, S. (1979) Psychopharmacology of mania. In B. Shopsin (ed.) *Manic Illness*. New York: Raven Press, pp. 177–218.

Silverstone, T. and Turner, P. (1982)* *Drug Treatment in Psychiatry*. London: Routledge and Kegan Paul.

Szasz, T. S. (1963) *Law, Liberty, Psychiatry*. New York: Macmillan.

Szasz, T. S. (1967) *The Myth of Mental Illness*. New York: Harper and Row.

8 Contemporary psychopharmacology: a review

D. J. Sanger and D. E. Blackman

In this concluding chapter an attempt is made to sketch a general picture of contemporary psychopharmacology, drawing in particular from the contributions to this book. This includes some consideration of the ways in which drugs can be used as tools to further our understanding of normal and abnormal processes at the behavioural, psychological or biochemical levels. This is followed by a brief consideration of some general methodological and even ethical issues in psychopharmacological research, illustrated by means of a general description of how new drugs are developed and brought into use, with particular reference to potential psychopharmacological agents.

Contemporary psychopharmacology

In Chapter 1 the reader was warned that psychopharmacology is a diverse area of study involving aspects not just of psychology and of pharmacology, but also of subjects as disparate as chemistry, medicine and sociology. The two major parental disciplines of this truly interdisciplinary field themselves present in their own right daunting challenges to their students: psychology studies the whole range of animal and human behaviour and experience by means of a battery of different empirical methods, while pharmacology has advanced in a more constrained and traditional scientific manner, to such an extent that it has achieved considerable mastery of detail with respect to its analyses of drugs and their effects on living materials. Any introduction to psychopharmacology must therefore be selective or illustrative, even perhaps idiosyncratic. Thus there are many areas of active psychopharmacological research and topics of general psychopharmacological interest which have not been directly addressed in the chapters of this book. The present selection has sought rather to illustrate the methods and scope of a field of endeavour which is inherently interesting to most people, which is currently vibrant, and which poses considerable challenges for empirical and conceptual analyses.

In Chapter 2, Barrett outlines research which is perhaps particularly marked by its objectivity and scientific rigour. The data discussed are those resulting from studies in which animals are exposed to carefully controlled experimental conditions. Psychologists have long used such methods to investigate how environmental circumstances can influence the behaviour exhibited by animals. Barrett's review of what is often now designated 'behavioural pharmacology' shows how research has established that principles which are important in understanding behaviour in its own right can also be important for an understanding of the behavioural effects of drugs. Whatever the direct biochemical or physiological effects of a drug might be, it has thus become clear that the effect which the drug exerts on overt behaviour can differ as a result of the experimental conditions controlling the behaviour. For example, the rate at which a pattern of operant behaviour occurs, which is largely the result of the environmental conditions to which an animal is exposed, can be an important determinant of the behavioural effects of stimulant drugs, influencing not just the size of any drug effect but even on occasion its direction. Barrett also discusses such other factors as discriminative control of behaviour, the nature of the event which maintains behaviour, and the prior behavioural and pharmacological history of an animal, all of which can exert powerful effects on the behavioural outcome of drug administration.

Of course the experiments discussed by Barrett may appear unduly constrained: their experimental control is bought at the cost of taking behavioural pharmacology into the narrow and artificial world of the laboratory and of studying as a model the behaviour of laboratory animals rather than that of people. Are such findings of any more general relevance in psychopharmacology, in the more complex circumstances in which people take drugs which affect their behaviour? This is of couse to a large extent an empirical question, although we may note that it is in general a traditional and successful strategy of scientists to create simplified and artificial models through which to study phenomena in controlled experiments, and they have often produced data which have proved to be of relevance to the less structured world outside the laboratory. It is claimed that the studies reviewed by Barrett identify some simple organizing principles which can be illustrated in controlled experiments but which may be of relevance to the real world. For example, Robbins and Sahakian (1979) have suggested that the apparently 'paradoxical' effect whereby hyperactive children become *less* active after the administration of psychomotor stimulant drugs may be an example of a rate-dependent drug effect outside the confines of the experimental laboratory. It will be recalled that high rates of lever-pressing by animals may be reduced by the administration of amphetamine, and this extrapolation of the principle of rate-dependency provides an example of attempts to extend the principles of experimental behavioural pharmacology with animals to the less structured world in which we live. It might also be noted in this respect that the rapid progress which has been made in recent years in biochemical pharmacology and neurochemistry is based almost entirely on laboratory studies with rats and mice.

The work reviewed by Stolerman in Chapter 3 is in the same general tradition as that discussed by Barrett. Controlled experiments with animals are used to investigate the ways in which drugs can act as stimuli, and thereby gain control over behaviour. The fact that drugs can serve as reinforcers in operant conditioning experiments with animals and thereby maintain behaviour may be of relevance to our understanding of situations in which drugs are abused by people (Griffiths *et al.*, 1980). Experiments in this area alert us to the possibility that different patterns of drug-seeking behaviour may emerge as a result of the ways in which the drug is scheduled to occur. Perhaps equally important, other events which depend on behaviour and which stand in some specified relationship to a drug may also exert a powerful influence over behaviour. The extrapolation of these principles to our understanding of drug addiction is discussed by Stolerman. Also of importance in his chapter is his discussion of how, in technical terms, drugs can come to serve as discriminative stimuli.

Such work may begin to address experimentally the question of the subjective properties of drugs, and it alerts us to the fact that drugs may come to exert control over behaviour if they stand in a specified relation to any non-pharmacological reinforcer. The principles to be extrapolated from such work are perhaps important to our attempts adequately to understand the general psychological as well as the pharmacological context of drug abuse, a problem in psychopharmacology which cries out for more sophisticated psychological analyses with which to supplement the established pharmacological methods of investigation. The latter, though detailed, seem not to identify unequivocally the conditions in which a substance will or will not be abused (Schuster and Johanson, 1981).

Chapters 4 and 5, by Lowe and Cochrane respectively, review work which focuses more directly on the effects of drugs taken by people in their social worlds and on the circumstances in which drugs are abused. Such an approach of course enjoys greater face-validity with respect to problems confronted by individuals and to more general social problems relating to drugs, and it also makes it possible to supplement behavioural data with direct reports of subjective experience when drugs are taken. Both chapters reveal that this approach to psychopharmacology can quickly lead to great complexity with respect both to the reliability of empirical findings and to the identification of explanatory principles. Lowe's discussion of the behavioural and psychological effects of alcohol and of alcoholism and its treatment illustrates such complexity clearly. Thus the effects of alcohol, whether studied in physical, behavioural or psychological terms, can be complicated by marked differences between individuals, by context-specific factors, and by such psychological features as expectancy. Such complexities become even more pertinent in relation to increasing our understanding of alcoholism and to our attempts to control alcohol abuse. It seems that alcohol can exert specific physiological effects, and this makes the search for physiological mechanisms potentially desirable and profitable. On the other hand, the effects of alcohol and the conditions in which alcohol dependence develops cannot be seen simply in physical or physiological terms. This illustrates practically the claim that psychopharmacology must be an interdisciplinary subject: the effects of alcohol depend on both pharmacological and psychological factors, and no doubt on interactions between these factors. Such a comment is, of course, reminiscent of the conclusions prompted by the experimental work with animals reviewed earlier. Exactly similar arguments can be made with respect to the effects on people of nicotine and smoking, where pharmacological and psychological factors also clearly interact. For example, although some have sought to emphasize the significance of pharmacological factors (i.e. nicotine) in cigarette smoking (e.g. Schachter, 1978), it is also clear that psychological factors are important in the development, maintenance and control of smoking (e.g. Frederiksen and Simon, 1979).

The use of alcohol and of nicotine is of course legal in Western societies. Cochrane's chapter extends the analysis to the use of illegal drugs. Cochrane emphasizes in particular the ways in which illegal drug use has been conceptualized in terms of *social* psychology. Perhaps in part because of the social contexts created by social disapproval and legal sanctions for the taking of drugs such as marijuana and heroin, his review of the evidence leads Cochrane to conclude that the explanation of marijuana use and even of heroin addiction in terms of social roles is more compatible with the facts relating to the taking of these drugs than are pharmacologically based explanations. This is not, of course, to claim that substances such as marijuana and heroin are pharmacologically inert (although the pharmacological effects of marijuana can sometimes seem elusive). The literature on the effects of both legal and illegal drug use leads inexorably on the conclusion that pharmacological and psychological factors are both relevant to an adequate understanding of the phenomena, and of course that these factors interact in both contexts. It is perhaps the social contexts of legal and of illegal drug use which prompt researchers to emphasize pharmacological or psychological factors to a greater or lesser extent, or indeed which prompt greater prominence for pharmacological or for psychological influences on drug-taking behaviour.

Chapters 6 and 7, by Smith and Harrison-Read respectively, consider the effects of drugs of greater potential significance in medical and therapeutic contexts. Smith reviews experimental studies of the effects of drugs on memory processes and clinical studies of the effects of drugs on disorders of memory. The experimental studies use human subjects, often in the context of theoretical models of information processing, and investigate the effects of drugs, many of which act upon cholinergic synapses. The conclusion that it is easier to produce evidence for drug-induced *disruptions* of memory in normal subjects than for enhancement may disappoint those who aspire to a pharmacological panacea to help us cope with the ever-increasing demands of our life-styles or improve our ability to process and retrieve ever more information. However, the clinical studies of therapeutic effects of drugs on memory disorders appear more encouraging, and the synthesis of experimental methods and clinical relevance appears particularly useful in this field, promising as it does to elaborate the specific effects of drugs on psychological mechanisms and even on the physiological or biochemical mechanisms underlying them. Currently there is a great deal of both basic and clinical research being carried out with the aim of discovering and developing novel drugs effective in alleviating cognitive problems in elderly patients. Although no drug has yet been accepted as unequivocally effective (Reisberg *et al.*, 1981), it is possible that significant new discoveries will soon be made (Bartus *et al.*, 1982).

Harrison-Read reviews the use of drugs in psychiatry. Clinical pharmacology has in general made significant contributions to medicine, to such an extent that one has almost come to expect that a drug be prescribed to ameliorate or cure any medical condition. It is therefore perhaps natural that many should hope for a similar contribution for clinical psychopharmacology, with respect to the amelioration or even the cure of behavioural and psychological disorders; and indeed drug treatment is by far the most widely used form of therapy for such conditions. In fact psychoactive drugs are among the most widely prescribed drugs for any medical condition. Harrison-Read's chapter places the hope for drugs effective in all mental disorders in its historical context in psychiatry, and reviews the effects of some of the drugs currently in therapeutic use. He also evaluates the ways in which drug interventions can be abused, and clearly does not advocate a psychopharmacological approach to therapy which takes no account of the variety of factors which can predispose individuals to mental illness. Once more this can be expressed in terms of the need to incorporate both pharmacological and psychological methods and explanations in the interdisciplinary study of psychopharmacology. It should be noted that clinical psychopharmacology can be evaluated merely in pragmatic terms, but Harrison-Read points out that the discovery by essentially pragmatic methods of effective psychopharmacological substances has in turn led researchers to develop and evaluate hypotheses which relate mental illness to putative underlying physical disorders.

The chapters in this volume, then, illustrate (but do not define) the methods and interests of contemporary psychopharmacology. Empirical enquiry in this field may be experimental in nature, using either animals or humans as subjects, may rely on the more analytic methods of social science in the empirical investigation of phenomena in the world outside the laboratory or clinic, or may relate directly to clinical conditions, principally in the hope of achieving therapeutic gain. It need hardly be emphasized here that none of these broad approaches is in any sense better than the others. Indeed, psychopharmacology is particularly rewarding as a subject partly because its very complexity demands an appreciation of the relevance of a wide variety of techniques. As a result, psychopharmacological research is sometimes able to offer a greater degree of synthesis between differing empirical approaches to its problems than psychologists have come to expect in their own domain. For example, experimental studies of the behavioural effects in animals of events associated with drug re-inforcers may make some contact with social psychological analyses of the context in which drug abuse develops or is sustained (O'Brien, 1975). In turn, these enquiries prompt more awareness of the complexities in the aetiology of drug addiction and a sensitivity to the requirements for a careful evaluation of therapeutic interventions. They may also suggest in turn some possible kinds of therapeutic intervention which may prove to be useful. To take a rather different example, essentially pragmatic studies of the therapeutic effects of drugs on memory disorders may prompt speculations about the physical substrates of the processes involved in memory. These speculations can be evaluated by means of sophisticated psychological studies of the effects of drugs on the various processes of memory in normal human subjects, and indeed by means of experiments with animals which may introduce the possibility of more direct manipulations of potential physiological substrates. Psychopharmacology is rich not just because of its combination of psychological and pharmacological subject matter, but also because it encourages the imaginative use of differing research strategies in an attempt to chart the effects of psychological and pharmacological variables and their interactions.

It is also perhaps worth re-emphasizing here that psychopharmacological research illustrates not just the combination of different research techniques but also the ways in which different levels of explanation can coexist or even complement each other. It has become increasingly clear that psychopharmacology cannot aspire to explanations of its phenomena couched exclusively in reductionistic terms of physiological or biochemical processes, although these are undoubtedly important. Explanations in terms of behavioural or psychological principles (such as those of rate-dependency, social role, or cognitive expectancy, for example) must also be accommodated. These different levels of explanation can sometimes more readily appear to be mutually supportive in psychopharmacology than is perhaps the case in psychology, a discipline dogged by schismatic debate about 'appropriate' levels of explanation.

Finally it is worth mentioning briefly that psychopharmacological research can sometimes be used to throw direct light on issues which are essentially either psychological or pharmacological in nature. This point is perhaps best illustrated here in general terms. First, drugs can sometimes be used to further psychological analyses: a drug which is clearly established, for example, as an effective anxiolytic may be used as a probe to investigate the contribution of anxiety to some behavioural performance (e.g. Gray, 1982). If anxiety is thought to be a necessary component of a learning situation with animals, for example, then administration of the anxiolytic drug might be expected to affect their performance in a predictable manner. Conversely, the use of well-understood psychological or behavioural procedures can contribute to the pharmacological analysis of a substance. Drugs can therefore be used as tools for the study of basic behavioural or cognitive processes and different patterns of behaviour can be used as tools for the study of the pharmacological activity of substances. Examples of both approaches can be found in the chapters of this book. It must always be kept in mind, however, that just as there is no pattern of behaviour which is at present completely understood, there is also no drug whose pharmacological effects are entirely specific at either the behavioural or the biochemical level.

Methodological issues and the development of new drugs

It has been emphasized above that psychopharmacology draws its data from a wide range of empirical enquiries. In this final section, some very general issues not previously discussed in this book are mentioned, particularly by reference to the stages in the development of a new therapeutic pharmacological agent. Such research and development is carried out almost entirely by commercial organizations motivated by the substantial profits which can be obtained from a true advance in effective pharmacotherapy. While some deplore the unashamedly commercial nature of this aspect of medicine (e.g. Klass, 1975) there is no evidence that an adequate level of funding could be maintained for effective drug development by any other system. Also, the testing and marketing of new drugs is closely monitored and regulated by government agencies in all Western countries. Indeed it has been suggested that the level of regulation is at present so stringent that it is leading to the discouragement rather than the encouragement of innovation (Weatherall, 1982).

Although there are currently many drugs available for the treatment of psychiatric disorders such as schizophrenia or depression, all have problems of limited effectiveness or significant side-effects. Thus, most psychiatrists seem agreed that there is a need for novel psychoactive agents with greater safety and efficacy. Therefore, many pharmaceutical companies are engaged in the search for such drugs. The stages in the development and production of a new drug in the United Kingdom have been discussed by Greenwood and Todd (1977), and are illustrated in Figure 8.1.

In pharmacology generally, the development of a new drug falls into several phases which normally extend over at least eight years. It should be emphasized that the success rate in developing new therapeutic compounds which can be marketed is extremely low. Greenwood and Todd (1977) claim that the Pharmaceutical Division of ICI in the UK alone tests some 8000 new compounds per year, of which only between five and ten may be selected for further development. At least half of these will in turn fail tests of safety evaluation pre-clinically. Only after successfully passing such tests can a drug be subjected to clinical trials, and these too of course will lead to the elimination of further substances. Thus Greenwood and Todd emphasize that the production of one major new drug every two to three years would indeed be a successful record for any pharmaceutical company. It should be emphasized here that these data relate to clinical pharmacology generally. One might expect the development of clinically useful *psycho*pharmacological substances to be even more hazardous from a commercial point of view, for it has been emphasized by all the contributors to this book that the effects of drugs on behaviour are sometimes difficult to classify and evaluate unequivocally and are multidetermined. Quantitative psychopharmacology certainly provides greater challenges than does the measurement of a specific

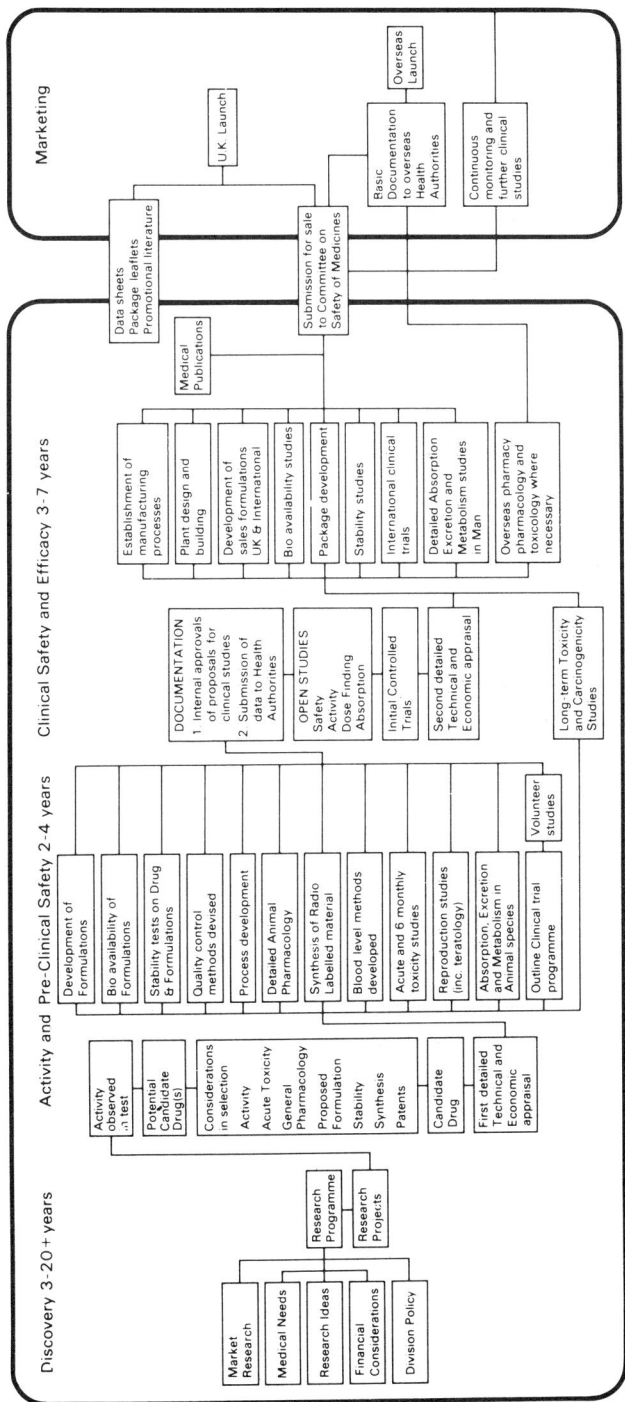

Fig. 8.1 Stages in the development and production of a new drug in the United Kingdom.

Source: Greenwood and Todd (1977).

change in some localized bodily system, such as the control of blood pressure for example.

In this brief review, the final stage of commercial development of a new drug, that of marketing, will be ignored, and no emphasis will be placed on the essentially chemical development programme which leads to the systematic production of new substances to be tested. Of greater importance here is the pre-clinical stage which evaluates the activity and safety of a new substance. Greenwood and Todd (1977) outline the general areas of investigation at this stage, and again only some of these are of direct interest here. For example, studies of how a substance can be produced effectively, how its quality can be controlled, how stable it is, how it may be formulated for clinical doses, and so on, do not have any biological content. However, there are a number of biological tests to which drugs being evaluated at this stage must be put. These include studies of the distribution, metabolism and excretion of the substance by animals, studies of blood levels of the substance, studies of toxicity and carcinogenesis, and studies of the effects of the substance on reproduction (teratology). To these must be added, of course, careful studies of the specific effects of the substance with respect to its intended use.

With respect to psychopharmacological agents, a number of behavioural tests with animals are usually included, in order to obtain a behavioural profile of the substance under investigation. The use of animals (normally mice and rats) as subjects reduces to some extent the ethical problems posed by the use of drugs whose effects are yet to be identified and whose safety is not yet established, though it should be emphasized here that there is of course a moral cost in subjecting animals to such procedures and such work is regulated and monitored in the United Kingdom by the Home Office. The requirements for building a behavioural profile of a drug's effects, as is the case with non-behavioural effects, tends to put an emphasis on simplicity and speed, in order that large numbers of animals can be readily tested. Observation of the general behaviour of test animals can yield useful information. Level of alertness, changes in the amount of motor activity, grooming behaviour or stereotyped patterns of behaviour, vocalizations and general bodily movements, the amplitude of startle responses to noise, motor co-ordination, urination and salivation, and changes in food and water intake are all reliably induced by specific drugs, and the profile of a new substance with respect to these tests may be compared to those of established drugs whose psychopharmacological effects are well known (Irwin, 1968). Thus, if the profile of a new drug on these tests is similar to that of an established antidepressant, for example, this may be taken as initial support for the possibility that the substance may itself have antidepressant activity.

These general tests can be supplemented by more specific tests. For example, analgesic drugs lead to longer latencies in the removal by rats of their paws from a hot surface or to a higher threshold of stimulation to the tail before it is flicked. Potentially anxiolytic drugs can be investigated in tests believed to induce a level of fear or anxiety in experimental animals and potential stimulants can be studied to identify their actions on locomotor activity. Some behavioural tests may build on possible interactive effects between a test substance and other drugs, a technique which is widely used in pharmacology generally. For example, prolongation of sleeping time induced by a barbiturate drug is characteristic of certain classes of drug.

Simple behavioural tests such as these, which are referred to as screening tests, can provide much information about the effects of putative psychopharmacological substances. The need for quick and simple tests has already been emphasized, and such tests may often prove reliable and effective discriminators between different classes of drugs despite their sometimes apparently low face-validity. Tests with greater behavioural sophistication, such as those using operant conditioning techniques, are of course available, but they are far more expensive in terms of time and laboratory resources. However, they may offer a degree of experimental control which can lead to a reduction in the large numbers of animals which are conventionally used in the less controlled tests outlined above, where experimental groups must be sufficiently large to allow statistical designs to deal with large individual differences between animals and with other forms of 'noise' in the data. They may also, through their greater sophistication, provide more reliable predictions of a drug's therapeutic activity. Thus, for example, punishment procedures such as those outlined in Chapter 2 by Barrett, can be used to assess the effects of possible anxiolytic drugs. It will be recalled that animals' reinforced operant behaviour can be suppressed or disrupted by punishment with noxious stimuli, and anxiolytic drugs reduce such disruptions. However, as will be clear from Barrett's chapter, the interpretation of such an effect is not without its problems: rate-dependencies or differences in discriminative control, for example, might make it difficult to relate unequivocally any reduction in disruption to the supposed anxiolytic effects of a drug rather than to other effects which it might exert. Nevertheless, despite such problems, there does appear to be a good correspondence between the ability of drugs to increase rates of punished responding in laboratory animals and their clinical efficacy in the treatment of neurotic disorders (Cook, 1982). Other possibilities from operant conditioning are discussed in Stolerman's chapter. For example, tests of the extent to which response-dependent drug administration reinforces operant behaviour are essential in the analysis of the effects of new analgesic or stimulant drugs with potentially addicting properties. Again, Stolerman mentions the possibility of using drug discrimination tests as part of a routine screening procedure for psychopharmacological substances (see Colpaert and Slangen, 1982).

Substances which emerge satisfactorily from the extensive biological and more specific behavioural evaluation procedures with animals may then be exposed to pre-clinical tests with normal human subjects. This stage brings with it further methodological problems. For example, the use of volunteer subjects is an ethical necessity at this stage, but the validity of research using volunteers has caused controversy in psychopharmacology and indeed in psychology generally. Volunteers may differ from the general population in many ways (on the basis of age, education, occupational status, personality, etc.), and any of these variables may produce a systematic distortion in pre-clinical trials, giving undue emphasis to some effects of a new drug or, worse, hiding other effects which may operate selectively on individuals in the community with different characteristics from those prominently represented in the experimental sample.

The experimental designs of pre-clinical investigations with volunteers (and indeed of subsequent clinical trials) must make due allowance for the expectancy effects outlined by Lowe and Cochrane in earlier chapters. Thus the expectancies aroused by the experiments may induce placebo effects which may distort experimental data in unspecified but systematic ways. The routine incorporation of placebo in this stage of evaluation does not necessarily of course eliminate such placebo effects: it merely, though importantly, makes it possible to identify the effects of a drug which are additional to any placebo effects induced by the experimental circumstances in which the drug is taken. The expectancies of the research scientists at this stage can also have a distorting effect on experimental data, but, because of the constraints operating on most volunteer trials, it is often considered impossible to use procedures in which neither the experimenter nor the subject knows whether a drug or a placebo is being used on a specific occasion (double-blind).

Only after all these stages, and as noted earlier only relatively rarely, is a new substance ready for clinical testing, when it can be introduced experimentally as a potential therapeutic agent for patients. Here it is essential that the drug be introduced in such a way that its effects can be carefully and objectively measured and un-ambiguously interpreted. Thus there is a need to control for placebo effects and to incorporate double-blind methods. Careful attention must be paid to appropriately designed experimental and control groups and clinical evaluations must of course incorporate carefully designed tests with unambiguous and objective dependent variables. The complexities of clinical testing have been well summarized by the various contributors to a book on this topic edited by Johnson and Johnson (1977). Special mention should be made here, however, of the ethical difficulties inherent in this stage of the process. By the time a drug has reached this stage, considerable evidence has of course been accumulated about its effects, both generally and specifically, both in animals and in human volunteers. There is thus a good deal of support for the view that the drug will prove useful clinically. It thus requires a high degree of respect for the demands of adequate empirical enquiry to decide on the one hand to allow some patients the chance to benefit from the drug while on the other hand denying this possibility to a similar group of control patients. It is generally believed that new drugs can be shown unequivocally to be effective only if they are tested in comparison with a placebo in double-blind trials. However, because of the ethical considerations it is sometimes thought undesirable to use a placebo, and a novel drug may be evaluated in comparison with a well tried and tested therapeutic agent in a study without a placebo condition. Such decisions about the design of clinical trials are not taken lightly, particularly where they involve serious mental disorders (Clayton, 1982). For example, in a trial in which a new drug is being evaluated for its effectiveness in treating depression, a decision must be taken as to whether the drug's efficacy can be compared with placebo in patients who might well be prone to attempt suicide without effective therapeutic intervention. The ethical implications of such a decision are obvious, yet there is a real sense in which we cannot be confident that a drug is indeed effec-tive unless we expose it to appropriate and sensitive evaluation.

The processes outlined above apply of course to the development of any new drug, not just those drugs which may have psychopharmacological properties. The review indicates some of the methodological and ethical issues in the development of drugs, but most of these are essentially extensions of issues in psychopharmacological research more generally. The use of animals in experiments raises questions about the extent to which data and principles may be extrapolated from controlled situations to the world in which humans live. In the case of commercial screening, however, the interests of quick and reliable screening techniques militate in favour of simple tests which may have little face-validity and against the systematic exploration of the behavioural variables which research has demonstrated can have such an important influence on the effects of any drug. On the other hand, the use of human volunteers in pre-clinical screening requires a sensitivity to psychological influences on pharmacological effects, although the problems of extrapolation from samples of normal humans and perhaps from artificial experimental laboratory situations to the putative clinical population should not be overlooked. Finally, the clinical trials emphasize yet again the need for carefully designed empirical studies if the behavioural effects of drugs are adequately to be identified and evaluated.

Conclusion

In this final chapter an attempt has been made to provide a modest integration of the materials discussed earlier. Thus the general research strategies in psychopharmacology have been juxtaposed of experimental investigations with animals, studies of the social context of legal and illegal drug use, and investigations of drugs with possible therapeutic effects in a psychological or behavioural context. The diversity of methodological approach complements the diversity of explanatory schemes necessary in contemporary psychopharmacology, for it has become clear from all these approaches that the psychological or behavioural effects of any drug are likely to be mediated not just by biochemical or physiological processes but also by those variables which are known to have behavioural or psychological significance generally. Within psychopharmacology, drugs can be used as tools to investigate any of these processes, but the most striking feature of contemporary psychopharmacology is its truly interdisciplinary nature. It draws empirical data from different methodological approaches, and is forced to give due weight to differing influences, psychological and pharmacological, on its findings. Such an interdisciplinary field therefore must build on the achievements and subtleties of its two parent disciplines, and not seek to reduce one to the other. The search for new and therapeutically useful psychopharmacological agents must recognize this, although at present development procedures tend to be more sophisticated with respect to the influence of pharmacological than of psychological variables. The brief consideration of how new drugs are developed, however, illustrates once more the diversity of research methodology in psychopharmacology, and it also serves to emphasize some ethical issues with respect to the needs of empirical enquiry in this field.

References

Bartus, R. T., Dean, R. L., Beer, B. and Lippa, A. S. (1982) The cholinergic hypothesis of geriatric memory dysfunction. *Science 217*: 408–17.

Clayton, D. G. (1982) Ethically optimised designs. *British Journal of Clinical Pharmacology 13*: 469–80.

Colpaert, F. C. and Slangen, J. L. (eds) (1982) *Drug Discrimination: Applications in CNS Pharmacology*. Amsterdam: Elsevier Biomedical Press.

Cook, L. (1982) Animal psychopharmacological models: use of conflict behavior in predicting clinical effects of anxiolytics and their mechanism of action. *Progress in Neuro-Psychopharmacology and Biological Psychiatry 6*: 579–83.

Frederiksen, L. W. and Simon, S. J. (1979) Clinical modification of smoking behavior. In R. S. Davidson (ed.) *Modification of Pathological Behavior*. New York: Gardner Press, pp. 477–556.

Gray, J. A. (1982) *The Neuropsychology of Anxiety: An Enquiry into the Functions of the Septo-Hippocampal System*. Oxford: Oxford University Press.

Greenwood, D. T. and Todd, A. H. (1977) From laboratory to clinical use. In F. N. Johnson and S. Johnson (eds) *Clinical Trials*. Oxford: Blackwell, pp. 13–35.

Griffiths, R. R., Bigelow, G. E. and Henningfield, J. E. (1980) Similarities in animal and human drug-taking behavior. In N. K. Mello (ed.) *Advances in Substance Abuse*. Vol. I. Greenwich, Conn.: JAI Press, pp. 1–90.

Irwin, S. (1968) Comprehensive observational assessment: 1a. A systematic, quantitative procedure for assessing the behavioral and physiologic state of the mouse. *Psychopharmacologia 13*: 222–57.

Johnson, F. N. and Johnson, S. (eds) (1977) *Clinical Trials*. Oxford: Blackwell.

Klass, A. (1975) *There's Gold in Them Thar Pills*. Harmondsworth: Penguin Books.

O'Brien, C. P. (1975) Experimental analysis of conditioning factors in human narcotic addiction. *Pharmacological Reviews 27*: 533–43.

Reisberg, B., Ferris, S. H. and Gershon, S. (1981) An overview of pharmacologic treatment of cognitive decline in the aged. *American Journal of Psychiatry 138*: 593–600.

Robbins, T. W. and Sahakian, B. J. (1979) 'Paradoxical' effects of psychomotor stimulant drugs in hyperactive children from the standpoint of behavioural pharmacology. *Neuropharmacology 18*: 931–50.

Schachter, S. (1978) Pharmacological and psychological determinants of smoking. *Annals of Internal Medicine 88*: 104–14.

Schuster, C. R. and Johanson, C. E. (1981) An analysis of drug-seeking behavior in animals. *Neuroscience and Biobehavioral Reviews 5*: 315–23.

Weatherall, M. (1982) An end to the search for new drugs? *Nature 296*: 387–90.

Name index

Figures in italics refer to bibliographic references

Allen, R. P., 146, 149, 152, *173*
Andersson, K., 155, *170*
Andima, H., 123, *135*
Antelman, S. M., 184, *198*
Atkinson, R. C., 141, *171*
Aycock, E., *55*

Baddeley, A. D., 142, 163, 164, *171*
Baez, L. A., 24, *53*
Bagley, S. K., *172*
Bailey, M. R., *173*
Bakker, C. B., *136*
Baldessarini, R. J., 191, *198*
Balster, R. L., 59, *82*
Balter, M. B., *137*
Banks, W. P., 89, *106*
Barnett, D. B., 160, *171*
Baron, M., 186, *199*
Barrett, J. E., 28, 29, 30, 41, 45, 47–52, 53–5
Barry, H. III, 24, *55*, 60, 63, *82*, 93, *106*
Bartus, R. T., 205, *215*
Bath, P. E., 130, *137*
Becker, H. S., 118, 120, *136*
Beer, B., *215*
Bennett, J. P., 14, *20*

Berger, P. A., 177, *198*
Bergner, L., *135*
Berie, J. L., *172*
Bigelow, G. E., *215*
Bjurstrom, H., *107*
Blachly, P. H., 127, *136*
Blackman, D. E., 3, *20*, 23, 33, 41, *54*, *56*
Blum, R., 116, *135*
Boulton, A. A., 12, *19*
Brecher, E. M., 114, 123, 129, *136*
Broadbent, D. E., 141, *171*
Brooke-Crutchley, J., 114, *139*
Brouwers, E. Y. M., 161, *172*
Brown, J. K., 130, *136*
Buschke, H., 143, *171*
Butler, M. C., 116, 117, *136*
Butters, N., 164, *171*

Caine, E. D., 147, 149, 150, 151, 152, *171*
Callaway, E., *108*
Cappell, H., 75, 92, *106*, 119, *136*
Cardozo, C., *54*
Carlin, A. S., 119, *136*
Cermak, L., 164, *171*

Subject index